Body Broken

The Church Needs the Great Physician

David Riley, MD

ISBN (Paperback): 979-8-9942306-8-8
ISBN (eBook): 979-8-9942306-7-1

Dedicated to Dad and Mom, faithful ministers to the Body of Christ throughout my life.

Table of Contents

Introduction

Those of us who are believers in Jesus are likely familiar with the fact that the Church is frequently referred to in the New Testament as the Body of Christ. In his letters, the Apostle Paul refers to this. At one point, he says 'You are the body of Christ, and each one of you is a part of it (1 Corinthians 12:27). In another passage, he refers to Christ being 'the head of the church, his body' (Ephesians 5:23). And yet again, he refers to 'Christ's afflictions, for the sake of his body, which is the church' (Colossians 1:24).

The human body is our physical presence in the world. It is what people see and recognize, and allows us to interact and communicate. When we think of a friend or relative, their physical form is what we picture.

Like our physical human body, the church as the Body of Christ is His physical presence in the world. We are to show people what He is like. When the world thinks about Jesus, they likely will picture aspects of Christians that they know.

Bodies come in many shapes and sizes. Consider various athletes. Marathon runners may be streamlined with very little body fat, whereas sumo wrestlers tend to the other extreme. A jockey may be small of stature, while some basketball stars are several feet taller. Each may have very different attributes that contribute to success or failure in their chosen pursuits.

In addition, our community has an influence on how our bodies interact. Cultures around the world impact how we dress, what we eat, and the sound of our conversations.

Likewise, local church bodies come in many shapes and sizes. Some are small house churches with fewer than twenty members, while others are large megachurches with thousands who join in worship. Around the world, different cultures impact styles of worship and ways of interacting with unsaved people around them. Some denominations emphasize various doctrines over others while still following Biblical teachings.

Despite these differences, the human body is designed to the same basic specifications wherever it is found. We have two eyes, ears, arms, legs, lungs, and kidneys. Our heart has four chambers and is in the middle of our chest. A doctor trained in America is able to capably treat an Aboriginal native in the outback of Australia, assuming they would allow it.

In the Body of Christ, despite the differences in congregations, each local body of believers has much in common. We trust the truth of God's word, believing the same orthodox tenets of our faith the world over. Worship practices may look and sound different, but will usually include songs of praise, participating in the Lord's Supper, water baptism, and giving of our resources to support the ministries of the church.

When functioning well, the various cells and organ systems work well in close cooperation. Our body can inhale air, extract oxygen, absorb it, and distribute it to all of our cells. We can ingest food, break it down, absorb the nutrients and vitamins necessary for our body to function, and excrete the unnecessary ingredients as waste. Our organs can filter the blood of toxins, regulate the heart rate and blood pressure, and maintain a consistent body temperature in almost all environments. And we reproduce in a complex and unexpected way that allows us to combine genetic material, ensuring diversity, producing another body that can do each of these things as well.

The main control center of our body is located at its apex, the fragile and convoluted brain, encased in bony armor for protection. It oversees the major functions of the body, maintaining its health and stability, ever vigilant to sense trouble and direct appropriate actions and movements to avoid danger.

When working well, the various members of the local church Body work well in close cooperation. We breathe in the presence of God, we receive the message that is delivered, we digest it to break it down, analyze, and hold onto the good stuff, disregarding the part we may not need at the time. The pressures we face are regulated through our interactions with fellow worshipers (i.e., organs) of the Body. We reproduce by reaching others, allowing God to deliver new spiritual life into the world.

The Body of Christ is ruled by the head (Christ) to direct our actions, help us avoid dangers, and sense trouble. The messages delivered come from Him through the spiritual leaders of each Body.

When first created, our physical bodies were designed to be perfect and to live in a perfectly created world. However, when Adam and Eve sinned, our bodies became susceptible to disease and decay that were not originally intended. From that point until today, everyone on earth has faced danger daily. God, in his omniscience, was prepared for this. He gave each of us an incredible ability to fight off disease and heal from injury. We truly are fearfully and wonderfully made, as David declared in Psalm 139:14.

Similarly, the Body of Christ was also created with health and strength. Many of us are familiar with the old hymn, and the words "'Tis a glorious church without spot or wrinkle. Washed in the blood of the Lamb." (By E. T. Rinehart, 1901). This is based on Paul's words in Ephesians 5:25-27. The context of this passage indicates that Christ loves the church and sanctifies and cleanses her with His word. This is what makes the church, His body, glorious, holy, and without blemish.

As we exist in this fallen world, both our physical body and the Body of Christ may suffer disease or injury. Although most of these ailments heal with time and treatment, some are more severe or overwhelm our ability to heal. These can leave behind scars or limitations in function.

This book will explore each of the main organ systems of our physical body and some of the problems that can occur. There are spiritual parallels in each system. As you read, I hope you will become familiar with the various 'disease processes' that can occur in the church. As we learn to recognize these deviations from the normal intended functions, we can take steps to correct them before they cause damage to the body. If we fail to identify these problems early, even small problems can grow severe enough to impact the ability of the body to continue functioning. This applies both to our physical body as well as the Body of Christ.

1

Complete Physical— Spiritual Assessment

2 Corinthians 13:5 "Examine yourselves to see whether you are in the faith; test yourselves. Do you not realize that Jesus Christ is in you—unless, of course, you fail the test?" (NIV)

Luke Wareham is here for a physical and wellness visit. He is 48 and has been in good health. His health insurance offers an incentive if he comes in for a checkup and labs. He does not have any specific health concerns.

Review of his history indicates no recent illnesses, no hospital stays, and no regular medications. He drinks alcohol on the weekends and does not exercise regularly. He does not follow any specific diet.

The examination is normal, other than his body mass index (a calculation comparing height and weight. The recommended goal is a BMI of 25) is 32, indicating obesity. His blood pressure is upper normal but acceptable.

Our discussion centers on improving his health. I tell him he needs to exercise and diet to improve his weight and blood pressure, and to limit alcohol intake as well. According to the guidelines, he is due for a baseline screening colonoscopy, so I order this for him. He is due for vaccines for influenza and tetanus. He reluctantly agrees to receive these. I order blood tests to screen for cholesterol, glucose, liver and kidney problems, and advise him to follow up in one year.

*****

Problems vs Prevention

The role of a doctor in many ways parallels the role of a pastor. In the medical office, our patients arrive with a variety of concerns and health problems. Many of them come in only when there is a problem that affects their daily lives, and we address the particular concern of the day. These visits may be infrequent. Even at a problem-focused visit, the doctor may try to address some long-overdue physical screening or preventive measures, hoping to improve the patient's overall health, therefore preventing more severe medical issues.

Other patients take more responsibility for improving or maintaining their physical health. They are more consistent in scheduling preventive physicals and following screening guidelines. At these routine visits, usually once yearly, we review the basics of their past medical history. We review healthy habits in diet and exercise. If they already have ongoing health struggles, we follow up on pertinent labs, treatments, and medication refills.

At all visits, it seems the doctor's primary role is to point out areas of the patient's physical health that could be improved. As the adage goes, nobody's perfect. There is always room for improvement, no matter how good someone's health is.

Similarly, in our spiritual lives, many people will come to church or talk to their pastor only if there are problems affecting their daily lives. Once that problem passes, they may not come again until another issue arises. Even at these infrequent visits, many if not all pastors will likely discuss the basics of a healthy spiritual life. They may emphasize the importance of spiritual activities, especially prayer, Bible reading, and Christian fellowship. Attending to these activities will help in preventing more severe problems in our relationship with Christ.

Others take more responsibility for improving and maintaining their spiritual health. They consistently attend church and engage in spiritual practices geared to improving their walk with the Lord. At these regular church services, the pastor addresses topics that may be basic for routine spiritual health, encouraging a healthy 'diet' of reading the Word and helpful devotional books, and 'exercising' by way of tithing, or serving others. There may be spiritual struggles specific to the local congregation or individuals, and the pastor can continue routine 'treatment' specific to these concerns.

As with our physical health, a primary role of the church leader is to point out areas of our spiritual health that can be improved. As noted in Romans 3:10: "There is none righteous, no, not one." The Lord Jesus, Himself, said "You shall be perfect, just as your Father in heaven is perfect" (Matthew 5:48).

In medicine, patients sometimes complain that the doctor is always negative, pointing out that they are overweight, scolding them for smoking, or engaging in unhealthy lifestyles. This can cause some to avoid coming in because they don't want to be judged or feel they are failing, although that is not the reason we address these topics. In church, even more so, people complain of being judged or condemned, when that may not be the pastor's heart at all. In fact, this sometimes may be the convicting work of the Holy Spirit. Unfortunately, it is an excuse used by many to avoid church as well as avoid those who call themselves believers.

It's Not Always Enjoyable

There are some aspects of a physical checkup that are not pleasant. Some of the questions I ask are personal. If the patient is not honest, it may hinder their ability to improve their health by denying some harmful habits or physical impairments and wounds. Portions of the examination can be more intimate, embarrassing, and awkward (for both the physician and the patient!). The recommended testing can be uncomfortable, for example colonoscopy, pap smear, or mammogram, but they can be very important in finding problems that need to be addressed before they become severe enough to threaten life or health. Vaccines are not fun, and no one enjoys having sharp needles in their arm, no matter how skilled the nurse may be at administering shots, but the benefits can be significant.

I have heard it said that spiritual leaders are tasked with not only comforting the afflicted but also afflicting the comfortable. It is true in the clinic as well. Many times, we need someone to challenge us, pushing us to improve. Things in our lives will not change unless acted upon by an external force, just as Isaac Newton proposed in his first law of motion (An object at rest will remain at rest unless acted upon by an external force). This applies to our physical health in topics such as exercise and weight loss. Doctors may seem to nag their patients on these topics at each visit. Spiritually, we feel a spiritual 'nudge' or conviction of the spirit to incite change in our lives.

Room for Improvement

I believe many of us spiritually are in a similar situation to this patient. We are in pretty good spiritual health, and we go to our 'checkup' each Sunday to get guidance on how to improve our condition and avoid problems in our spiritual life. We all have areas that we can improve. Some of us have become lazy in our walk with Christ, and we need more spiritual exercise, whether that be areas of service in our local congregations or being intentional in displaying our faith in the workplace. Our diet is not what it should be. We like our spiritual junk food of quick half-page devotionals and cultural or topical sermons. We prefer to keep things superficial, and we bristle at messages that would require us to step out of our comfort zone. We need to be encouraged to delve deeper into the meat of the word, and sometimes to hear tough talk about areas in which we lack strength or maturity.

If we are not willing to let God's spirit examine every aspect of our lives, we will continue in unhealthy spiritual habits and develop spiritual wounds that won't heal. The majority of the time, this will require that we set aside our pride and be open with God about even the most embarrassing or shameful thoughts and behaviors. There may be times we need to do uncomfortable things like going forward for prayer in a public service or giving up things that we enjoy so we may achieve better spiritual health. The promptings and convictions of the Spirit may sometimes be sharp and uncomfortable, like a vaccine, but will ultimately guide us in ways that will help us avoid spiritual shortcomings and failures.

The Schedule is Subject to Change

In my office, we schedule appointments based on what the patient indicates they need for the visit. When I get to the office in the morning and review the list of appointments, I tend to plan my day and formulate an idea of how each visit will go before I even start. Many days, however, there is something that changes the schedule. A patient listed for a physical may have a heart arrhythmia or a symptom they did not mention that requires more aggressive attention or hospital admission. If this occurs early in the day, the entire schedule can then be disrupted. I confess, I get easily frustrated if my vision of how the day will progress is changed, and falling behind can cause me to get irritable.

Similarly, our pastors plan each sermon series, many times months in advance, and develop a vision for the church week by week, month by month. Although this plan is ideally developed with prayer, we must hold that plan loosely. God may have another plan or may intervene unexpectedly. Church members may have more severe or acute spiritual needs that they kept to themselves. Once these are confessed, they need attention and prayer support from pastors or church members, and the schedule must change. I have fond memories of church services where the Spirit fell over the congregation even before the sermon was preached. God worked in the lives of many people as altar calls, and prayer times were extended. Lunch was delayed while fractured relationships were mended.

In this electronic age, we program our services to the appropriate length, but we must be willing to give all of that up as God directs. Our spiritual health depends on letting the Great Physician intervene when and where He desires.

Summary

No one has perfect health, either spiritually or physically. We all can benefit from regular examinations and preventive measures. Regular evaluation of our physical status is important in guiding us to proper health. Identifying diseases early allows us to treat them quickly before they cause damage to our body as a whole. Spiritually, regular involvement in the fellowship of the local church encourages us to better spiritual health and allows the Lord to identify spiritual problems before they take root and damage not just our own souls but the larger Body of Christ.

What's in a name?

Luke Wareham is lukewarm in his approach to health habits, both physical and spiritual. He is neither cold nor hot. In Revelation 3:15-16, Jesus speaks to the Church of Laodicea, stating:

> "I know your works, that you are neither cold nor hot. So then, because you are lukewarm, and neither cold nor hot, I will vomit you out of My mouth."

Being spiritually lukewarm is not a good place to be. It is a place of poor spiritual health. Regular 'checkups' can guard against this.

A. The Clinic: Where the Body Goes

A common phrase in Christianity is that the church should be more like a hospital (or clinic) for sinners than a museum for saints. Some may feel they must behave in a certain way or give up things they enjoy in order to be a part of the church. If they see someone in the church lapsing into sin, or having an angry outburst, or any number of things with which they disagree, they are quick to call out hypocrisy. The truth is that all of us who believe understand that we are sinners saved by grace. We are defined by our belief and surrender, not our behavior, but as we mature in our faith, the behavior follows.

If the same opinion held true in the medical world, only healthy people would go to the doctor, and they would be very judgmental of those sick, weak individuals who ask for treatment. It is the one who admits to needing help that comes in for evaluation and then can improve.

If the doctor is obese, it may hurt his or her credibility. However, doctors are human beings subject to disease. Even flawed, sick doctors can offer care and treatment to their patients. In the same way, pastors are subject to the same temptations and struggles as their congregation. But God specializes in using flawed people to reach a hurting world. It is His power that saves, not the talents or strengths of humans.

I see many similarities between the church and a medical clinic. Throughout this book, we will explore comparisons between the facilities and organizational structures of each. You will find a new facet of this discussion after each chapter.

2

Skin—Our Appearance to the World

Ephesians 5:25-27 "… Christ also loved the church and gave himself up for her to make her holy, cleansing her by the washing with water through the word, and to present her to himself as a radiant church, without stain or wrinkle or any other blemish, but holy and blameless." (NIV)

Sarah Eisess is 63 and is here for a rash. She was working in her yard pulling weeds three days ago, and the next day began to have red, itchy welts on her forearm. Yesterday, it was on both arms and became more blistered with some weeping of yellow fluid. Today, it has spread to her abdomen and legs as well as a few spots beginning on her face. She is miserable from the itching, and Benadryl and calamine lotion offer no relief.

On examination, she is afebrile (i.e., she does not have a fever), but her blood pressure is a little high. She appears uncomfortable as she tries to keep herself from scratching by rubbing her arms across her abdomen. There are red blistered-appearing lesions on her skin that have yellow-tinged fluid weeping from them, and some are crusted. The left arm has several of these lesions arranged in a line, but she also has similar spots on all four extremities as well as the back of her neck. Smaller red spots are noted on her face.

Her history and exam are consistent with exposure to poison ivy. The itching can be severe and may spread from one area to another as the skin reacts to the oils from the plant. This reaction does not usually stay localized, but it is not spread by scratching or touching the spots (assuming the oils have been washed off the skin).

I order a cortisone shot and a steroid pill pack and recommend she continue to treat the itching until it improves. She should be back to normal in a few days.

*****

When a patient schedules an appointment for a 'rash,' that can mean just about anything on the skin. If it is a child who also has a fever, viral illnesses are a common cause. Strep throat can lead to 'scarlet fever' with a sandpaper-like rash across the abdomen. Anyone could have an allergic response, whether to medicine or food, or other offending agents. Hives can come and go for many reasons, and sometimes we can't identify the cause. Psoriasis is a lifelong problem with areas of thick silvery scales and plaques, and eczema can cause dry itchy skin of variable severity that comes and goes depending on allergies or cold weather. Shingles may be very painful, but it is only on one narrow part of the body. And on and on. Even anxiety and worry can manifest on the skin.

Several of the skin problems referred to above can have parallels in the church. Just as the skin is what others see when they look at us, spiritual 'rashes' mar the appearance of the church. Let's explore a few possible causes.

Contact Dermatitis

As the name describes, this is skin inflammation (dermatitis) that occurs in response to contact with a triggering agent. Sometimes this can be localized, showing itself physically as a single patch of red irritated skin that may be specifically shaped to the offending agent. For example, an adhesive bandage (band aid) can leave two red square patches separated by a clear space where the adhesive contacts the skin in susceptible people. Or a reaction to a new eye-shadow can sometimes lead to red, swollen eyelids. Poison ivy is a similar reaction, but it does not stay localized. It may spread to many areas of the skin across the body. Generally, the best approach is to avoid the substance that causes the reaction. Once it is present, the dermatitis can be slow to resolve, but usually will respond to a steroid medicine. Generally, if someone has a sensitivity to a specific substance, this reaction will continue to occur throughout life.

Similarly, some in the church have a sensitivity to certain topics or behaviors and become judgmental or angry, sometimes lashing out with inflammatory words or expressions. This can be very noticeable to those outside the church and can be experienced as exclusion and alienation.

Just as each patient may have different sensitivities, believers can have triggers that vary from person to person. Someone growing up in an alcoholic family may appear more judgmental to those who drink, or someone betrayed in marriage may show a magnified response to those who have been involved in broken marriages or sexual sin. Sometimes this is localized in the body to one believer whose response is not shared by the church as a whole. However, this can sometimes spread to others who are susceptible to being influenced or who are not as mature in their relationship with Christ.

It is wise to separate ourselves from those things that cause an initial emotional response that can be off-putting. Ideally, we do not want to pull back from interfacing with the world, but if we have a human emotional response that pushes others away, limiting contact can be helpful while we allow the Lord to work on that aspect of our lives. Although physically the skin's tendency to react will be with us throughout life, spiritually, there is a cure. As we mature in our faith and our walk with Christ, His Spirit can temper those responses. As we produce more of the fruit of the Spirit, we are visibly more loving, joyful, peaceful, patient, gentle, and on and on. As with all spiritual maladies, the cure is a closer walk with Christ.

Infections

Viral illnesses can cause a variety of rashes on the skin, but generally are self-limited. The childhood vaccines for measles, mumps, rubella, and chicken pox can prevent several of the more dangerous illnesses, but there are many others that, although less dangerous, are still contagious. Some viral skin conditions, such as warts, may be ongoing until they are destroyed. Bacterial skin conditions, like impetigo or cellulitis, are many times more contagious and can spread until treated appropriately. I will discuss infections later in this book.

Shingles

Zoster, or shingles as it is commonly known, is an interesting rash. Typically, it is very painful, and sometimes the pain precedes the visible outbreak. It occurs along the distribution of a single nerve, so it manifests itself as clusters of blistered and crusted spots in a narrow band on one side of the body where this nerve functions. It will not cross to the other side of the body.

It is caused by a reactivation of the chicken pox virus, varicella. When we had chicken pox as a child, the infection may have cleared, but the virus remained. It lay dormant, like a sleeper cell waiting to be activated to terrorize the body. The trigger may be difficult to identify. Some patients can point to a specific physical or emotional stress or to recent treatment with a steroid that may lower resistance. Many do not have an identifiable cause.

The active rash of shingles may last up to two weeks and then slowly heal. Occasionally, it leaves behind visible pigmented spots that persist. One troublesome risk is post-herpetic neuralgia, a chronic burning nerve pain that may remain for years. The incidence of this painful complication increases with age, to as much as twenty percent in those over eighty years old.

If shingles occurs on particular parts of the face, it is possible for it to affect the surface of the eye, leading to scarring and possible blindness. Thankfully, this is rare.

Similarly, in our spiritual lives, we may have an offense from our past, perhaps from many years ago, that lies dormant. Maybe it was the time someone made an off-hand comment about us that hurt our feelings, or maybe we were not publicly honored for something we were a part of in the church. Each of us may have different things that are painful memories we have buried. Many times, we recover from this in a short time, but in some circumstances, it may leave a lingering emotional pain that simmers just below the surface for years.

Then, in response to some trigger that sometimes we can't identify, all the emotions and painful memories flare. The pain may be severe, preventing us from our usual function in the Body of Christ. It potentially could even blind us to spiritual truths. Over time, the noticeable effects of 'spiritual shingles' (the 'rash,' if you will) fade, and we are able to hide our pain from those around us. However, the pain may remain severe for many years, and if we continue to hide our pain, it will fester.

In order to rid ourselves of the chronic pain of 'spiritual shingles,' we must bring these inner struggles and painful experiences out. Talking to a trained counselor or a trusted member of the Body of Christ allows us to process these topics in more healthy ways, healing our hurts as we mature in our faith.

Physically, we may be able to prevent shingles with a vaccine. The spiritual 'vaccine' would be to deal with these past hurts before they cause pain and interfere with our role in the Body. Once again, we need others in the Body to help us identify healthy ways of processing hurtful experiences before they hamper our spiritual health.

Just as shingles physically is localized to one small segment of the body, 'spiritual shingles' is usually isolated to an individual hurt and does not spread to other members, although our pain will many times impact our interactions with others. It is true that 'hurt people hurt people.' Physically, there is no good treatment other than time and pain control. Spiritually, our hope for healing lies in trusting God with past hurts that we cannot change.

Birth Marks

Although technically they are not rashes, many people come to see me with concerns about skin spots. Parents may bring in their child to look at a birthmark. These are usually just blemishes on the skin in various shades of pigment. Many are pale brown or light tan, but occasionally they can be bluish black. Most are on areas of the body that are inconspicuous, but at times they may elicit comments from others. There are cases where the blue-black shades of some birthmarks have been mistaken for bruising, raising suspicion of abuse. Others, like hemangiomas that are related to tangles of blood vessels, can be large and angry-looking. Port-wine stains are, as the name implies, maroon-colored lesions that can be fairly large and may cover one side of the face or one extremity.

In general, birthmarks do not require any intervention. However, the more visible lesions on a child's body can lead to bullying or mocking by other children, or comments that cause hidden emotional scars. These may need to be surgically treated with laser devices or other specialized treatments. This procedure may be scary and requires the parent (as well as the child, if they are old enough to understand) to consent to the treatment.

Spiritually, our souls are all marked from the time of our physical birth. We refer to this as original sin. God's perfect creation was forever marred by sin when the Fall occurred as described in Genesis chapter three. Scripture is clear that "All have sinned and fallen short of the glory of God." None of us can cure ourselves of this stain on our souls. Thanks be to God that He is our cure. We do not need lasers or surgery. The blood of Jesus cleanses us from all unrighteousness. When we begin our new life in Christ, we are born again, leaving behind the spiritual marks from our first birth. As Paul said in 2 Corinthians 5:17 "…if anyone is in Christ, he is a new creation; old things have passed away; behold, all things have become new."

Acne

Most of us have acne at some point in our lives. Generally, this occurs as a response to the hormone changes of puberty. Although it is a normal stage of life, we all feel awkward as we endure this. Many relate this to their diet, blaming it on chocolate or greasy foods. The shelves of the pharmacy are filled with a myriad of ointments and solutions offered as treatment for acne. When these fail, the family doctor or dermatologist has plenty of other treatments that can be prescribed. Ultimately, most of us leave this condition behind as we leave our teenage years.

Spiritually, when we are young in our faith, we may display several awkward blemishes as we suffer the growing pains of maturing in our walk with Christ. We may remember with some embarrassment the spiritual opinions we held as babes in Christ. As our souls' diet advances from milk to solid food (as noted in

Hebrews 5:12-14), our faith matures. Our appearance before the world changes as these spiritual pimples fade away.

Summary

Our skin is the appearance we present to the world. It is how we are recognized. In John 13:35, Jesus said all will know we are His disciples if we love one another. Love is our 'make-up.' Just as physically some cover blemishes with 'concealer' or other products, 1 Peter 4:8 says love will cover a multitude of sins.

We want to be 'attractive' in the sense of drawing others closer to Christ. It is true, none of us is perfect or flawless. However, Ephesians 5:25-27 tells us Christ loved the church (the Body) and gave Himself for her that He might present her as a glorious church, not having spot or wrinkle or any such thing, but that she would be holy and without blemish. This is not something we can do ourselves, but it is the sanctifying work of Christ in His Body, the church, which improves our appearance.

What's in a name?

Our fictional patient is Sarah Eisess. This is a reference to psoriasis, a chronic skin disease that causes thick silvery scales and plaques on the skin. It is incurable but can be controlled with various medications and even ultraviolet light treatments. This is one of the few times tanning can be helpful to the skin.

B. The Clinic: Symbols and Affiliations

When someone is sick or suffering, they come to the clinic (or urgent care facility, or hospital) to get care. Some clinics have small storefront locations, some are large multispecialty buildings or hospitals. Each has different capabilities depending on size, budget, and personnel. Usually, these buildings are clearly marked, some with identifying symbols that are recognizable despite which hospital group or company operates them. This may be a red cross or a blue 'H' sign on a highway exit. Many will recognize the 'snake on the pole' symbol, whether it be the two-snake Caduceus or the single-snake Rod of Asclepius. All of these may signify a clinic or urgent care where sick people can get the care they need to restore health.

Similarly, the physical church facility has several characteristics to identify it. Almost all church buildings will have the symbols of our faith, be it a cross or maybe a dove, or angels. I need not remind you that the 'snake on a pole' medical symbol has probable connections and definite similarities to the incident noted in Numbers 21:4-9. Verse 9 notes:

"So Moses made a bronze serpent, and put it on a pole; and so it was, if a serpent had bitten anyone, when he looked at the bronze serpent, he lived." (NKJV)

This was also referenced by Jesus in John 3:14:

"And as Moses lifted up the serpent in the wilderness, even so must the Son of Man be lifted up, that whoever believes in Him should not perish but have eternal life." (NKJV)

In this parallel, we see that when people are physically afflicted (not necessarily by snake bites, but that could apply as well), if they look to the 'snake on a pole' of medicine for treatment, they can receive care. Spiritually, when we are afflicted, looking to Jesus lifted on the cross we receive healing of our souls. The symbols on our buildings guide us to the care we may need.

In addition to the more general symbols of healthcare, there are several well-known healthcare corporations spread across the country now. These organizations that are flourishing with multiple locations have their own branding to identify them, and patients can expect a similar style and level of treatment when they go to these locations. In my area of the country, we have hospitals that are part of the Hospital Corporation of America, or HCA system, and throughout the country, there are Kaiser Permanente hospital locations. The Veterans Administration provides care to military veterans all over the country. My own local hospital system was recently merged with our local university hospital system, which has locations all across our state. In each case, their branding and corporate policies are intended to be standardized across the organization, making their facilities recognizable and the patient experience more uniform between locations.

Similarly, our many church denominations may have their own branding and logos. The doctrine and bylaws of each denomination help to ensure that Baptists who attend Baptist churches in different locations will have similar worship experiences, while Nazarenes in various locations will find similar songs and educational materials, and worship experiences as well. Each denomination may differ in their worship style or doctrines while still following Christ.

Even within each system, whether it be medical or religious, individual doctors or pastors may have a personal approach or emphasis that falls well within the orthodox practices or doctrines. Both medicine and ministry incorporate the personality and style of the care provider.

On the other hand, some clinics are independent and not affiliated with corporations. Most of the time, these still provide proper standards of medical care, but without the accountability brought by oversight and bylaws of the larger corporation, there is a higher risk that an individual doctor may have treatments and beliefs that are more on the fringes of usual care. Some may emphasize vitamin infusions or sell supplements. Some focus on less common conditions that may not be as prevalent as the treatments they dole out.

Likewise, independent churches, for the most part, serve God and preach the Bible appropriately. However, without the affiliation with a larger denomination, there could be more risk of unorthodox beliefs and practices (snake handling, perhaps). This requires discernment and knowledge of scriptural truth for each of us in our worship.

3

Musculoskeletal Complaints—Structure

Hebrews 12:12-13 "Therefore strengthen the hands which hang down, and the feeble knees, and make straight paths for your feet, so that what is lame may not be dislocated, but rather be healed." (NKJV)

Ray Diaz is 17 years old and comes in with pain in the right wrist. He was playing basketball last night and was fouled, falling on his outstretched arm. He had immediate pain and, within a few minutes, noticed swelling of the wrist as well as bruising. He was unable to continue playing. The athletic trainer placed him in a wrist splint and advised he see us for further care. As I enter the room, he is sitting on the exam table, cradling his right arm. The arm is in a Velcro splint. On exam, he has significant swelling of the wrist. He has good sensation in his fingers and is able to move them, but this movement elicits pain in the wrist. He is hesitant to attempt flexing or extending his wrist due to pain. I order an X-ray, and it shows a non-displaced fracture of his radius. I place him in a short arm cast for six weeks, and then will follow up to repeat the X-ray.

*****

Musculoskeletal concerns are common in my office, whether it be teenagers playing sports, or weekend warriors doing household projects they are not physically prepared to do. Although there can be many causes for pain in the bones and joints, they generally fall under three simplified categories: they can burn out, wear out, or blow out.

Overuse injury (burnout)

Most of us at one point or another have developed sore muscles from doing a new exercise or sport, or from overexertion. This may become severe and greatly limit our ability to function until it has a chance to heal. As we use muscle tissue in ways in which it has not yet adapted, the small muscle fibers can break down and lead to muscle injury. The healing process lays down new muscle to reinforce this area so it will be ready for future use. As we continue to use the same muscles in the same way, we adapt and eventually suffer less pain.

I well remember the first time I went skiing. After falling numerous times and sliding down the bunny slope on my back repeatedly, I began to get the hang of it. After a couple of days, it was fun! But then, the pain kicked in. After a long car ride back home from Colorado, I arrived home to discover that I was almost physically unable to climb the stairs. I had overused the muscles of my legs and back in ways they had not been used throughout my lifetime. It took several days for the healing to be complete. Since then, I have skied without the need for such prolonged recovery as my muscles were better prepared.

Spiritually, we run the risk of overexertion as well. We may volunteer for positions in the church for which we have not taken the time to fully prepare. We can feel overwhelmed, and this may elicit pain in the form of frustration or hurt feelings. This may cause us to pull back and take time to recover, but when asked to serve again, it may spur us on to be better prepared.

Some in the church feel it is a spiritual duty to serve, and God may use each of us in various capacities. It is wonderful to serve, to volunteer, to teach, or whatever we feel led to do. There is a risk that those who are willing to step up may be asked to do so over and over again in many more areas of service. This 'overuse' of one member of the Body can lead to burnout. After a time, we are exhausted physically and emotionally. Spiritual fatigue may set in as well. For some, this may mean we just need time to step back and refresh our souls, but some become angry and bitter.

Setting proper limits and boundaries can help prevent such problems, and it is important for both individuals and leaders in the church to be accountable in honoring these limits. This is a spiritual truth that can be found in Creation, where God rested on the seventh day (Genesis 2:2). It is mirrored in the fourth of the ten commandments as we are told to keep a sabbath rest from our work. And Jesus tells us "Come unto Me all you who labor and are heavy laden and I will give you rest." (Matthew 11:28). We must care for ourselves in order to effectively care for others, finding a proper balance between service and rest.

Arthritis (wear out)

Our bones, joints, and tendons are susceptible to accumulated damage throughout our lifetime. Constant weight bearing and pounding of the knees with exercise can damage the protective layer of lubricating cartilage that covers the bones. Stress points can lay down extra calcium and form bone spurs. Injury may cause a piece of articular cartilage to break off and become a free agent, floating around in the joint and getting stuck at various points. As the damage accumulates, the healing process innate in our cells is unable to restore the tissues to pristine condition, leaving a buffet of symptoms. As we age, our joints may pop and grind or be stiff and swollen. Pain may accompany even simple activities. The medicines we use to treat such changes can slow the damaging processes but not reverse them. The pain can be controlled, but the medications could potentially lead to stomach ulcers or kidney problems. Certain joints can be surgically replaced, providing significant improvement in function, but still never back to normal.

Spiritually, as we age, we sometimes allow ourselves to get set in our ways, and spiritual stiffness can set in. Even someone sitting in our pew at church can be irritating and hard to accept. Friction points can lead us to be callused and have 'bone spurs' that cause pain when we must interact with certain people or situations. We can groan with any spiritual activity. This stiffness and pain primarily hurt us more than those with whom we interact, and our usefulness in ministry is limited. The forward progress of the Body, the church, can be hampered and slowed.

For all of us, our humanity can make us susceptible to these limitations, but scripture tells us in 2 Corinthians 4:16, "Even though our outward man is perishing, yet the inward man is being renewed day by day." The fruit of the Spirit will smooth all of our interactions if we humble ourselves and let Him do his work in and through us. Most of these troubles have more to do with being focused on our own needs than on the needs of others. When we become followers of Jesus, we enter everlasting life at that moment, and there need not be wearing down or aging of our spiritual joints.

Breaks and Tears (blow out)

Disruption of any tissue can be painful and debilitating, whether it be a fracture of a bone, a tearing of a ligament, or rupturing a tendon. The location of this trauma determines the severity of the disability and how long it may take to heal. Some of these injuries are severe enough to require surgical correction, and some can be life-threatening, depending on the structures they impact.

Fractures come in a wide range of severity. Small chip fractures of our fingers are painful but not dangerous or likely to cause problems after they heal. However, a shattered compound fracture (protruding through the skin) can lead to dangers of infection or blood clots, or even loss of a limb. Some fractures are subtle enough that we can continue to deal with the pain for days or weeks before we finally have it checked. Others require immediate emergency attention.

Orthopedic surgeons employ a variety of power tools to repair the damage done, and extended stays in rehab hospitals may be needed for certain injuries. Many people return to full activity, but future X-rays will always show evidence of a healed fracture line. Sometimes the enlarged knot of the bony callus can be felt under the skin. The more severe fractures will heal but leave some impairment of function, whether it be a permanent limp or an angled finger. Atrophy of the surrounding muscles may result if function is not restored quickly.

Just as fractures are signs of failure in the physical structure, spiritual fractures can be seen as a failure of the leadership framework in the church. Some of these may be hidden and localized, like a board member with anger control issues or a hidden drinking problem. Others can threaten to disable a church for a time, like blatant and visible moral failures. Whether it be sexual misconduct or financial embezzlement or some other misuse of power, these 'fractures' in the leadership cause the Body to come to a standstill.

Progress is halted, and the pain can be far-reaching. Church attendance may atrophy. Many times, the leaders need to be removed from their place of ministry to allow healing. Thankfully, God will bring healing in even the worst situations if we are willing to participate in the recovery process.

In cases of moral failure, especially when they become publicly known, there may be a profound impact on those who have been blessed through the ministry of those at fault. Recently, a world-renowned Christian speaker, defender of the faith, and author of many books passed away. Shortly after his death, word spread that he had been accused of sexual misconduct. Those who assumed leadership of the ministry that bore his name pledged to conduct an independent and thorough investigation into the allegations and to be transparent with the results. Shockingly, the accusations were found to be true.

I struggle with this. If I listen to one of his messages and grow in my faith, and then days or weeks later hear of his moral failure, does that mean there is no truth in the message? Surely the truth of God remains true even when the messenger is sinful. We know that we all have sinned and fallen short, but as a wise friend pointed out, God can draw a straight line with a crooked stick.

Imagine another man of God in a position of leadership who is caught in a lustful embrace, which leads to an unplanned pregnancy. The young lady is married to a man under his leadership. This leader attempts to cover his sin by giving this man time off work, hoping their marital activities will hide the source of the pregnancy. However, he declines this opportunity, wanting to serve in his responsibilities with his team. This "man of God" in leadership then orchestrates the man's death, hoping it will look like an accident. Here we have lust, infidelity, deceit, abuse of power, and murder, and yet this man, King David, is still known as a 'Man after God's own heart', as Paul quoted in Acts 13:22. David wrote many of the Psalms that bring us such deep comfort. Jesus himself quoted Psalm 22 while nailed to the cross.

In this day of anonymous Tweets and social media posts, many in the church are quick to condemn anything associated with leaders who have sinned. Books are withdrawn from bookstores, and podcasts are deleted. Imagine if David would have lived today. Would we still have some of the beloved psalms we quote?

I realize public sin needs public repentance. This recent spiritual leader died before this happened, and it appears he displayed an ongoing track record of engaging in this sin. My struggle is with the fact that his messages were so impactful before this was publicized. It is not him that we follow but Jesus, and his messages influenced many to follow the Lord.

We must consider the words of Paul in Philippians 1:18: "But what does it matter? The important thing is that in every way, whether from false motives or true, Christ is preached. And because of this I rejoice."

I realized many are hurt by revelations like this. It is so very difficult to separate the message from the messenger. Our spiritual leaders are held to a higher standard of behavior due to their role in the kingdom of God, and rightly so, but we forget that they are also sinners in need of a savior.

Of course, these 'injuries' will never destroy the church. Jesus said He would build His church and the gates of Hell would not prevail against it. His victory over evil is assured, even amid our ongoing battles.

Summary

Our physical structures, such as bones and muscles, allow us to stand and move in the world, protecting our vulnerable internal organs. Injuries to our structure require time to heal, and depending on location and severity, may require time away from normal daily activities or even hospitalization and surgery. In more severe cases, we may never move as smoothly and painlessly as we once did.

Spiritual structures are primarily those in leadership roles at various levels. Failures of the spiritual structures in the Body of Christ also cause varying degrees of damage and impairment that may require limited time away from duties in the Church body or possibly removal from office or some form of discipline by the governing board of the Church.

No matter the individual failures of our leaders in the Church, God has promised that He will build His Church, and the gates of Hell will not prevail against it.

What's in a name?

Our patient for this chapter is Ray Diaz. This, of course, refers to the radius, one of the bones that comprise our forearm. This bone extends from the elbow to the base of the thumb. Its structure at the elbow is reminiscent of a golf tee, and it is much thicker at the wrist. It functions along with the ulna, the other forearm bone, in allowing rotation of our wrists in pronation and supination (turning the hand palm down or palm up).

C. The Clinic: Layout and Equipment

Visit any medical clinic, and there will likely be many things they have in common. Usually, there is a reception area (aka waiting room) and a desk with receptionists who greet you as you arrive to help you prepare for the visit. Then a door leads to the larger area of the office where the care will be provided. The exam room will likely have unique furniture that people do not typically have at home, like an exam table and a wheeled stool. Some rooms may have more specialized furnishings, such as a procedure table or ceiling-mounted lights that are adjustable. If you were to stumble into the clinic unexpectedly without seeing the sign, you would still likely recognize it as a medical facility.

Similarly, churches tend to have common features throughout the country. There is probably a lobby with a welcome desk. Someone there is able to give information to prepare you for the service. Doors lead into the sanctuary, where there is furniture not typically found at home, such as church pews and a pulpit. The windows are likely to be more ornate, possibly stained glass. The raised platform at the front is not a stage for performers (although some may use it as such) but a place of proclamation that can draw attention to the message being delivered.

In the medical setting, once a patient reaches the clinical area, he may be exposed to several items of medical equipment that are possibly strange or unknown. They are unique to the medical environment. Larger clinics and hospitals typically have an X-ray machine that needs a shielded room, or Oxygen nozzles in the wall for quick access. Electrocardiogram machines are usually on a wheeled cart that can be moved from room to room as the need arises. Especially in the emergency room, the 'code cart' is a common item, usually red and on wheels with many drawers, like a fancy tool cabinet found in some garages.

In the exam room, the nurse taking the vital signs will likely check blood pressure using a sphygmomanometer, more commonly known as a blood pressure cuff. Many times, they will use an oximeter on the finger to measure oxygen content as well as heart rate. The nurse and the doctor may use a stethoscope to amplify the subtle sounds of the heart or lungs. Special lights are used to look in the ears (otoscope) and eyes (ophthalmoscope).

Likewise, in the church, we use various items in worship that are uncommon in other settings. It was common in the past to have a large organ, or a built-in baptistry in many churches. As mentioned earlier, there may be an ornate large pulpit that is not just a basic podium. A communion table is still present in many churches. The altar rail at the front of many sanctuaries may seem odd to the unchurched, and the baptistry is not just a hot tub but has a special and holy purpose. Many churches use shiny communion service sets that I have not seen in other contexts. Small glasses, stackable trays with many circular cutouts, and a tray with little pieces of hard bread could appear confusing and odd.

There is a trend in many churches to have chairs instead of pews and no pulpit on the platform. Organs may be replaced by electronic keyboards, guitars, drums, or, at times, even banjos. The built-in baptistry in some locations is replaced by a portable water tank or hot tub brought in for special occasions. Many locations have screens on the walls to show the words to worship songs, or information on upcoming events, or the pastor's sermon notes. Sound systems with speakers and connections in the walls or floor of the platform bring to mind the built-in oxygen or suction systems noted in clinical facilities.

Throughout the centuries, worship styles have changed and have been modernized while still holding true to the Bible. As practices are updated, equipment may change, but it still serves to advance the health of the Body of Christ. Change can be helpful to take us out of our habits and cause us to have a new experience, possibly encountering God in a new way. Even while changing, the environment is usually recognizable as a place of worship.

4

Kidney Function—Discernment

1 Thes 5:21 "Test all things; hold fast what is good." (NKJV)

Lupe Henley is 67. She comes in today because she is fatigued. She has not felt well for months, and for her general aches and pains, she has been taking high doses of ibuprofen. She has not had a checkup for many years, but remembers that last time her doctor said she had a problem with her kidneys. This scared her so she did not go back, and she has tried to ignore these symptoms ever since. Her daughter finally forced her to make the appointment. On exam, her blood pressure is very high (173/102), and her body mass index is 38. Her heart rate is elevated at 104, but is regular. She has edema in her legs and moves stiffly as she walks to the examination room. Her labs come back showing her potassium is high at 5.8, and her creatinine is 3.5 (more than twice the upper limit of normal), indicating kidney failure. Her urine is very concentrated, and analysis indicates it contains protein and blood. I refer her to a nephrologist, who determines that she has hypertensive nephropathy (kidney disease due to her uncontrolled blood pressure). Her use of ibuprofen is also damaging her kidneys. She eventually requires dialysis.

*****

The kidneys are amazing organs. Since they are so resilient in their function, most impairment in kidney function is temporary. This can be from dehydration, low blood pressure, blockage by a stone, inflammation from infection, or a variety of other sources. In most cases, hydration and time, along with relieving any obstruction, will allow the kidney function to return promptly to normal with no residual problems. However, repeated insults to the kidney will eventually cause a breakdown in the function of the fragile capillary filtration system that maintains our body's status quo. Eventually, it is possible to overcome the redundancy in the function of our twin kidneys and require outside help.

Filtration

One of the primary functions of our kidneys is to filter the contents of the blood and excrete impurities. They regulate the levels of electrolytes and vitamins, and many of our medicines are processed and excreted in the urine. They also maintain proper acidity of the bloodstream by adjusting the absorption and excretion of various molecules. They maintain blood pressure control and fluid balance. For diabetics, an excess of sugar is flushed out with the urine. Although our bodies can function with just one kidney, we have two to maintain function in case one of them is impaired.

Dialysis machines are man-made filters designed to approximate the function of our kidneys. They are lifesaving to many people, but they can never equal the efficiency and ability of our natural kidneys. Dialysis is generally not a good long-term solution. Transplant of a suitable donor kidney is much better, as long as there is good compatibility between donor and recipient to avoid rejection.

In 1 Thessalonians, Paul instructs us to test everything and hold on to what is good. This is an accurate description of a major function of our kidneys, and in the Body of Christ, we need that constant analysis as well. Spiritual discernment is vital to keeping the health of the church strong. Wrong doctrine or teaching that is not supported by scripture can lead us astray. This may lead to more pressure among the congregation, or caustic (acidic) criticisms of others.

We must know scripture well if we are to compare the truth of each message to the truth of God's word. Although our pastors and leaders may be more fully equipped for this function due to their education and training, all of us have a responsibility to learn. We should follow the example of the Bereans in Acts 17:11 who "... received the word with all readiness, and searched the Scriptures daily to find out whether these things were so." In so doing, we can hold our leaders accountable to teach scriptural truth.

Stones

At times, the minerals in the urine accumulate and form a stone. When these small stones travel from the kidney down the ureter toward the bladder, they can cause severe pain and blood in the urine. They may get lodged in the ureter and cause swelling and dilation as the urine backs up, causing pressure to the kidney. With increased fluid intake, we may be able to flush the stone through to the bladder so it can be passed, but many times it takes surgical intervention to retrieve the stone and place a stent in the ureter to offer protection while it heals.

At times, there may be spiritual blockages in the church. Some may hold stubbornly to erroneous ideas or teachings or be very strict in their judgements. These attitudes may block the function of some aspects of the church. Until this stubborn approach is 'passed' and repentance occurs, this can cause significant pain and be toxic to the body.

Physically, if a stone is too large to pass, a common technique of treatment is lithotripsy. Technically termed Extracorporeal Shock Wave Lithotripsy, abbreviated ESWL on patient charts, this involves sending powerful sound waves through a bath of water in which the patient is positioned, blasting apart the stones so the smaller fragments may then pass. For stubborn spiritual 'stones,' using not sound waves but sound doctrine can break down those faulty beliefs that are impairing the body.

Hydration

One of the best ways to protect the health of our kidneys is to stay hydrated. Drinking adequate water each day allows the extraction of more impurities from the bloodstream through the elaborate filtration system of the kidneys. Adequate hydration keeps the urine diluted so minerals are not concentrated enough to allow a stone to form. When we become dehydrated, the kidney suffers and function declines.

Similarly, our spiritual health suffers if we do not have adequate Living Water provided by our Lord. As we daily commune with God through the work of the Holy Spirit, Jesus promises "whoever drinks of the water that I shall give him will never thirst. But the water that I shall give him will become in him a fountain of water springing up into everlasting life." (John 4:14). This process of spending time in the Word of God, learning truth, leads us to knowledge in scripture and proper doctrine. In this way, our discernment increases and allows us to recognize untruths.

In times of spiritual dehydration, a long drink of Living Water can restore our souls. As we continue to fulfill our function of discernment, it can keep harmful teaching out of circulation in the church and help keep balance in function to keep the church strong. In cases where the church has lost its discernment, it no longer functions as it should, and error is compounded. At this point, it may take a transplant of new leadership with the necessary discernment to eradicate toxic beliefs and restore health to the body.

Summary

Our kidneys constantly analyze the contents of our blood, regulating the levels of electrolytes, acid, fluid, and impurities. This testing and filtering keep our body in balance physically to allow each of our organs to function as it was designed.

In our spiritual lives, the function of analysis and filtering is referred to as discernment. Each of us individually should be regularly learning from our leaders as well as from our own reading and Bible study, but not just taking everything we read at face value. As we learn, we are to test everything in light of the scriptures, and in so doing, we will grow stronger in our spiritual health, strengthening the health of the Body of Christ.

What's in a name?

Our patient in this chapter is Lupe Henley. In our kidneys, the Loop of Henle is the hairpin arrangement of collecting tubes that allows the concentration of certain chemicals. This allows urine to be collected and sent downstream to the bladder, where it is eventually expelled from the body. This is yet one more example of how intricately we are created.

D. The Clinic: The Exam

Many providers, including me, go through a similar process with each patient. We take the history of what is going on, telling us the reason for the visit. We review the medicine list and the past medical history. We do our physical exam in a standard order, and I must confess, sometimes I go through this routine without paying conscious attention. There are times after an exam, I have to stop and think, "Did I hear a murmur?" or "Did I already look in her ears?" and have to repeat what I just did as I pay more attention. We get set in our habits, and even if the patient supplied certain information to us already, we end up asking them for the same information because it comes next in our 'script.' After that, we formulate a plan and discuss next steps and things to work on.

Similarly, our church services often follow a well-worn path. We begin with a certain number of worship songs, followed by announcements, offering, prayer, and then maybe a responsive reading. The sermon is of standard length, and then there is a closing prayer and a song. Possibly an altar call or discussion of next steps and things to work on.

Through the years, many churches have moved away from liturgy or more formal worship. Weekly responsive readings or quoted blessings from the pulpit, or a standard pre-prayer song, may become habitual. As we experience this, week in and week out, we may grow desensitized to the wonder and majesty of it all. We sing familiar songs while our minds wander. Updating our worship and leaving behind certain rituals may serve to freshen our experience.

C. S. Lewis discussed this idea of liturgy or standard worship practices and had a different take on it. He states that the structure is meant to free us up to worship. Writing about worship structure, he states:

"…it "works" best…when, through long familiarity, we don't have to think about it. As long as you notice, and have to count the steps, you are not yet dancing but only learning to dance…. The perfect church service would be the one we were almost unaware of; our attention would have been on God." (Liturgy, found in *The Joyful Christian*, p. 80., c. 1977, MacMillan Publishing Co).

A little later, in the same essay, he talks about trying novel things in worship, with the result that we are distracted, wondering what is going on. I know for myself, a new song in worship can kidnap my attention as I try to figure out the words and the tune instead of listening to the message of the song.

I need to work on disciplining my mind and heart to focus on worshipping God, whether there are familiar comfortable aspects of the service or new ways to focus on Him.

5

Gastrointestinal—Processing the Message

Hebrews 5:13-14 "For everyone who partakes only of milk is unskilled in the work of righteousness, for he is a babe. But solid food belongs to those who are of full age, that is, those who by reason of use have their senses exercised to discern both good and evil." (NKJV)

Perry Stalsis is 39. He comes in with complaints of stomach pain accompanied by bloating, belching, and heartburn. It started two months ago, but he has been taking over-the-counter antacids, hoping it will resolve. Recently, it has worsened, and now at night he wakes up choking with an acid taste in his mouth.

On physical examination, his vital signs are normal, but his body mass index is 48, indicating morbid obesity. He admits to unhealthy dietary habits and drinks alcohol several times per week, as well as several cups of coffee each morning. He has tenderness in the upper abdomen just below the ribs.

I diagnose him with acid reflux and start him on a proton pump inhibitor. I also counsel him on lifestyle changes to reduce this problem, including weight loss, and avoiding caffeine and alcohol. Within seven days, he reports control of these symptoms.

*****

Our gastrointestinal (subsequently referred to as GI) tract is complex. It functions, in some ways, as a reverse assembly line, digesting and breaking down our food, rather than assembling a product. The journey begins in the mouth, where the food we ingest is crushed by our teeth into smaller fragments, as our saliva produces certain enzymes to start the digestive process. It descends through the esophagus to our stomach, where strong acid further breaks down our food.

From the stomach, it passes into the long tunnel of the small intestine. In the first portion, called the duodenum, pancreatic enzymes break apart protein molecules and release sugars, while the pancreas also produces insulin in case the sugar levels rise too high. The gallbladder secretes bile that has been produced in the liver, which further dissolves nutrients, especially fats, from the remains of our lunch. As the journey continues, these nutrients are absorbed through the lining of the intestines into the thin-walled capillaries, similar to the arrangement in our lungs that allows oxygen absorption.

Once it reaches the large intestine, also known as the colon, there are few nutrients remaining. As it journeys through the colon, water is reabsorbed, and the remaining material moves to the rectum, where it is eventually excreted, in the same way a kitchen juicer separates the healthy liquid juice from the remaining pulp, ejecting it.

Taste

I find it interesting that we have a sense of taste. Physically, this seems unnecessary since we are capable of taking and processing nutrition without it. For unfortunate patients who are unable to take oral food, they receive nutrition by way of a tube placed directly into the stomach, or temporarily through intravenous nutrition. This can be a drab existence and may lead to depression. Although taste may not be necessary, it adds great enjoyment to the act of taking in nutrition.

There are different types of taste divided into sweet, salty, sour, bitter, and savory (also known as umami). It is postulated that these help us identify dangerous substances such as poisons, and also may allow us to seek out those nutrients our physical body needs as we crave certain foods.

Spiritually, we are told to "Taste and see that the Lord is good." (Psalm 34:8). Elsewhere, the Word says, "For the ear tests words as the palate tastes food." (Job 34:3). These passages speak to 'tasting' the Word in the form of evaluating and considering its truth, not just blindly accepting everything we hear from our spiritual teachers. Beyond merely testing and evaluating, though, we have joy in our relationship with the Lord. We taste and see that He is GOOD! He is not just providing bland spiritual calories. The Psalmist says, 'How sweet are Your words to my taste, sweeter than honey to my mouth:" (Psalm 119:103).

At times in our spiritual lives, we may need to be reminded of certain spiritual truths. Even as we read familiar passages of scripture, we can 'taste' new things that strengthen and revive us. Just as we may at times developing a craving for certain tastes physically, the bible reminds us to 'desire the pure milk of the word, that you may grow thereby, if indeed you have <u>*tasted*</u> that the Lord is gracious." (1 Peter 2:2-4, NKJV, emphasis mine).

Acid Reflux

As food passes through the esophagus into the acid bath of the stomach, the lower esophagus has a circular muscle, a sphincter, that is designed to tighten and keep the acid from ascending into the esophagus. As noted in the fictional patient above, when acid trespasses into the esophagus, it can cause heartburn. If the acid remains there long enough, it may lead to ulcerations of the esophagus or narrowed, scarred areas of stricture that could prevent food from passing through this tight region.

Spiritually, God uses all kinds of personalities. Some people, strong believers and followers of Jesus, are more caustic in their personality or communication style. I liken them to gastric mucosal cells that produce acid and are adapted to the low pH of the stomach. Alternatively, many of us in the church are accustomed to mild-mannered, kind, humble methods of teaching that are very careful to avoid offending others. These are more 'esophageal mucosal cell' people, not designed for much exposure to acidic, caustic individuals.

There is a place for strong personalities that fearlessly address uncomfortable subjects, more concerned with truth than ruffled feathers. I believe the apostle Paul probably had that type of personality, since scripture clearly shows how many times people took offense at his bold teaching and plotted his death. Even Jesus did not pull any punches in his criticism of the teachings of Pharisees and Sadducees, calling them a brood of vipers or whitewashed tombs.

In more modern times, one Christian personality that comes to mind is Dr. Tony Campolo. I have no doubts about his Christian walk, but he has had a way of shaking some people out of spiritual stupor. One story that made the rounds years ago was that as he was speaking from the pulpit, he made the following statement:

> "I have three things I'd like to say. First, while you were sleeping last night, 30,000 kids died of starvation or diseases related to malnutrition. Second, most of you don't give a [s#&!]. What's worse is that you're more upset with the fact that I said '[s#&!]' than the fact that 30,000 kids died last night." (www.premierchristianity.com/Past-Issues/2015/July-2015/Holy accessed 3/17/2021. This quote was spoken during a sermon in 1982.)

I can only imagine the effect those words had on those listening, but the message is profound. Just as acid is physically necessary to break down our food to help with the digestion process, sometimes we need spiritually to break through our comfortable church life so we see past our assumptions to what may be more important.

I don't believe we should make this type of message the norm, however. Just as acid physically can cause burning and discomfort or even damage when it is in the wrong place, especially when it is there for too long, this type of prodding or 'afflicting the comfortable' can leave us burning with anger, or if prolonged, cause damage to a congregation.

Pancreatitis

Once the food passes from the stomach into the small intestine, the digestion process continues. The pancreas produces digestive enzymes that further break down the material to release nutrients. Sometimes the pancreatic enzymes begin to attack the wrong tissue leading to pancreatitis. This causes abdominal pain and vomiting with each meal. Depending on the severity, this may lead to chronic changes in the pancreas, reducing its effectiveness.

'Spiritual pancreatitis' may occur when educated people in the church, proud of their theology, use that knowledge to belittle or criticize others (as is commonly seen in social media comments).

This spiritual pride is hurtful and may lead some to have doubt or painful responses to each spiritual 'meal.' As this painful emotional response continues, even to good Biblical teaching, they are not able to grow spiritually due to these past painful experiences.

Malabsorption

Some physical conditions leave us with rapid transit of the digested material. These patients develop malabsorption syndrome, where the vitamins and nutrients that remain are not absorbed properly. This can lead to cramping and frequent diarrhea, which, if severe, can cause dehydration. This may be the result of various causes, including celiac disease or surgery to remove part of the bowel.

Spiritually, if we do not take time to meditate on what God teaches us through a sermon or Bible reading, it is quickly out of our heart and mind, and we gain no spiritual growth from it. God reminds us to 'be still and know that I am God' (Psalm 46:10) and also tells us that 'those who wait on the Lord shall renew their strength.' (Isaiah 40:31).

Constipation

Conversely, as the remnants of our diet pass through to the colon, there may be a very slow transition, and things get backed up. Too much water is reabsorbed, leading to constipation and more difficulty passing what is left. When this is more severe, it is called obstipation and can lead to intestinal blockage, decreased appetite, pain, and sometimes vomiting.

Similarly, in our spiritual lives, it is sometimes good to spend time meditating on one passage of scripture or aspect of our walk with Christ. However, if we focus on this to an extreme level, and get 'stuck' on this longer than the Lord intends, we can hamper our usefulness.

Summary

Our gastrointestinal tract allows us to take complex nutrients in our food and break them down so they can be absorbed and used. Each stage of our digestion plays a part in this. In a similar way, in our spiritual lives we 'feed' on messages containing complex doctrines and we need to be able to 'digest' these concepts. When we analyze and learn these truths, we are able to strengthen and nourish the Body of Christ. As we develop greater understanding, we grow and mature, and our diet can move from 'milk' to 'meat,' as referred to in Hebrews 5 in the verse noted at the beginning of this chapter.

What's in a name?

Our patient this time is Perry Stalsis. The term peristalsis refers to sequential muscle activity in the wall of a tube, which propels material through it. Medically, if this action is absent, it is called achalasia, and our food just sits in the esophagus. This causes a traffic jam that leads to increasing symptoms of heartburn and discomfort in the chest as the esophagus becomes uncomfortably stretched. Another condition may occur if we ingest something noxious. In that case, our stomach senses the problem and does an 'about-face,' sending it back where it came from. This is called reverse peristalsis, whereby the stomach contents are forcefully ejected (i.e., we puke).

E. The Clinic: Clothing

In the medical setting, there are certain uniforms and styles of dress. In the past, scrubs were generally worn by surgical specialists or obstetricians during procedures. Gradually, they began to be worn more consistently. Now, nurses and receptionists also wear them, many times coordinating the color of the scrubs to designate their role. Some doctors choose to wear the traditional long white coat. If a patient is undergoing a procedure or is admitted to the hospital, they get their own special outfit—usually a gown that hangs open in the back and has snaps securing the sleeves at the shoulders to allow quick removal during an emergency. During certain procedures, the medical team wears sterile gloves and masks as well. (Of course, during the recent pandemic, masks and gloves were not just for clinics anymore.)

In some churches, they still wear traditional uniforms. The pastor or priest may wear formal robes when preaching, and the choir may have gowns that match. In days gone by, even the congregation traditionally would dress in their Sunday best to go to God's house. Now, many churches do not follow this tradition, and the pastor and worship team may dress casually in jeans and tennis shoes. This is not all bad. It removes the pressure on some to appear a certain way and may break down barriers to a small degree.

One aspect of proper dress deserves more attention. When it is time for surgery, much attention is given to maintaining a sterile environment. Surgical infections can be a severe complication, and prevention is key. The patient is in a gown, and for abdominal surgeries, they may need to have hair removed around the site of the operation. Once in the operating room, powerful cleansing scrubs are used that are bactericidal, and everyone wears head coverings, masks, and shoe covers. Anyone involved in the procedure will also have sterile gowns and gloves, and prior to entering the operating room, will undergo a ritual of scrubbing for a certain amount of time, cleaning under the fingernails, and letting the water drip down off the elbows instead of possibly contaminating the already sterile hands. The scrub nurse holds the sterile gown up for the surgeon to thrust his hands into the sleeves, and then holds the gloves open for him to put his scrubbed hands in them. Once this is accomplished, the gown ties are carefully handed to a non-sterile tech without any touch of the sterile gloves, and the surgeon twirls around to then grab the sterile part of the tie to secure the gown. It is a carefully choreographed dance that occurs in all hospitals daily. The patient is then covered in sterile drapes to limit exposure to just the surgical field and avoid contamination.

Spiritually, there is a type of 'proper dress' not seen with the eyes. In Matthew 22:1-14, we read the parable of the marriage feast. The king invited guests to his son's wedding, but they were not willing to attend. Therefore, he sent out invitations to anyone who would come, and the wedding was filled with guests. Each guest was supplied with a wedding garment, but when the king saw a man who did not have on a wedding garment, he ordered him bound and cast into outer darkness.

When we become Christians, we are clothed in the righteousness of Christ. It is not supplied by our efforts but rather by our King. He invites us not out of our worthiness, but out of His own grace. 1 Peter 1:3 tells us, "His divine power has given us everything we need for a godly life through our knowledge of him who called us by his own glory and goodness." The next verse indicates that through His gifts we "may participate in the divine nature, having escaped the corruption in the world caused by evil desires."

I see this mirrored in the operating room. The surgeon and the patient are covered in 'garments' not their own, supplied for them. Through the wearing of these garments, we escape 'corruption' or contamination. If the surgeon scrubs with the correct scrub solution and brush and wears a freshly laundered outfit he picks out from home, he is likely cleaner than most people in the hospital. However, does being cleaner than everyone else mean he is clean enough to operate? Of course not. He needs the cover of the sterile gown and gloves due to his natural bacterial burden. In the same way, we can do good things and righteous acts all day long and count ourselves better than most others, but still not be good enough. Our sins need to be covered by the blood of Christ to impart the righteousness we must have to enter heaven.

Analogies naturally break down at some point. I do not see heaven as a sterile place where God is so weak and immunodeficient that we could contaminate Him with our unrighteousness. He needs no protection from us. In some ways, it is more like we are entering an infectious disease research facility 'hot zone' where deadly pathogens are present. We require full coverage and special diligence to protect ourselves. God's righteousness and holiness will pass judgment, annihilating the unrighteous, just like the man in the parable who did not wear the proper garment and was cast into darkness. If we leave any part of our lives uncovered, trying to keep back something for our own, that is susceptible to judgment, just like if we leave part of our skin uncovered in the pathogen lab, we are susceptible to deadly disease.

Only total surrender and the complete coverage of our sins by the blood of Christ will save us.

6

Reproduction—Evangelism

John 4:35b "Behold, I say to you, lift up your eyes and look at the fields, for they are already white for harvest!"

Inda Metrium is 52 years old. She comes in with hot flashes that are uncomfortable and disruptive. Intercourse has become more painful as well. She states the symptoms started nine months ago and cause her to frequently feel flushed, break into a sweat, and wake her from sleep. It has reached a point where her husband moved to the guest room. Her last menstrual cycle was over a year ago.

On examination, her vital signs are normal, and her body mass index is 27. There are no significant findings on her physical examination. The blood tests show low estradiol levels, confirming menopause.

Since she has no family history of breast cancer and gets regular screening mammograms, she is interested in starting estrogen replacement. I write the prescription for her to take daily.

She calls back in four weeks, reporting she feels much better, and the hot flashes are almost completely gone. Her husband moved back into the bedroom, and now she is requesting a sleeping pill due to his snoring.

*****

In our physical bodies, our ability to reproduce depends on numerous factors. For women, several different hormones must rise and fall at the proper time to prepare the uterus for, as well as to maintain, an early pregnancy. Men require certain hormonal as well as circulatory factors to play their part as well. These processes naturally decline with age. For women, the ovaries cease producing estrogen at adequate levels, leading to cessation of the normal monthly cycle of uterine preparation. As estrogen levels fall, there are other common effects on the body, including vasomotor flushing, otherwise known as hot flashes. Vaginal tissue begins to atrophy, leading to dryness and painful intercourse. Bone density is not supported to the same degree, leading to possible osteoporosis. And many other effects may occur.

For men, the testosterone levels may naturally fall, leading to decreased libido as well as difficulty achieving or maintaining certain bodily functions needed for reproduction.

In our society, sex is emphasized (some would say overemphasized) so much that many people feel they lose their identity if this part of life is taken from them. This has led to a huge market for pharmaceutical products for men as well as women to allow ongoing sexual function.

While women cannot regain fertility after menopause since ovulation is no longer possible, there have been cases where post-menopausal women have been given hormones to maintain a pregnancy conceived by in vitro fertilization of donated eggs. The oldest on record as of this writing was an Indian woman age 74 (https://www.oldest.org/people/oldest-person-to-give-birth/, accessed 9/27/2025), whose children were born in 2019. (Yes, children, plural! She gave birth to twins after in vitro fertilization with her husband, age 82. She had been ostracized in her community for not having children.)

Men, on the other hand, may continue to produce reproductive cells until death. There are numerous cases of men over 80 who have fathered children with their much younger wives. The oldest recorded in the past century was an Indian man, aged 96, with his 52-year-old wife (https://www.oldest.org/people/fathers/ ; accessed 9/27/2025), breaking his own record after he fathered his first child at the age of 94. The news media are fond of publishing reports of famous people, especially actors, who father children in their advanced age.

In our confused society, there are more and more same-sex couples who are not satisfied with adopting children but instead seek out procedures to allow them to become pregnant. There have even been famous stories about the 'pregnant man,' Thomas Beatie, who was born female and transitioned to male (including surgery). His wife was unable to conceive so 'he' had artificial insemination and had four successful pregnancies.

Sex and the desire to reproduce are powerful forces in our lives.

So, what happened to the spiritual body? It seems we have lost our spiritual 'libido,' our desire to 'reproduce' as we witness to others and bring forth 'baby Christians.' We have been commissioned by our Lord to 'Go and make disciples' in Matthew 28:19. Many of us, faithful Christians for many years, remain in our churches soaking up the sermons and never sharing the good news. Did something change since Jesus gave His disciples that instruction prior to his ascension?

Even for those who are more outgoing in sharing our faith, I believe many of us spiritually reach a time in our lives when we feel the torch has passed to a younger generation, and we can now retire and rest. However, I do not find that idea in scripture. Many of the heroes of the faith were called late in life to a new adventure of obedience.

In the Body of Christ, there is no 'spiritual menopause' or natural loss of fertility. We can and should be active participants in the Great Commission until God calls us home.

The Bride

In addition to the church being called the Body of Christ, scripture also refers to us as the Bride of Christ. He pursues a relationship with us, wanting spiritual intimacy and desiring to care for us. Our attentions are elsewhere, however.

You may be familiar with the popular television reality show franchise, The Bachelor, with its companion show, The Bachelorette. The premise is that one young woman, The Bachelorette, is designated for the season, and then twenty or more potential suitors are chosen from a large pool of applicants. The goal is for them to 'find love,' and the expectation is that at the end of the season, there will be a marriage proposal. Week by week, the Bachelorette weeds out the pool of men, sending home those who don't make the cut, until only two or three are left. The viewing audience thrives on the arguments, tears, and drama as the season progresses.

In many ways, we, the Church, are the Bachelorette. Christ pursues us, but we are bombarded by many other 'suitors' vying for our attention in this world. These suitors may include popularity, monetary success, pleasure, or a sense of self-importance. As we grow spiritually, the hope is that we shed each of the false suitors and choose Christ. To the world watching, unfortunately we in the church may display the same variety of drama, arguments, poor choices, and infighting that are commonly seen on the TV show.

Problem Relationships

As human beings faced with a variety of relationship choices, many times we choose poorly. Spending too much time in close relationship with the wrong people may lead to a variety of unwanted consequences, not the least of which are sexually transmitted infections. Some of these, such as herpes, have no cure and may flare up throughout our lifetime with painful outbreaks. Others, like HIV (the human immunodeficiency virus which causes AIDS), may work slowly, quietly, to decimate our health, reducing our immune system's ability to fight infections.

Other poor relationship choices may hurt us emotionally, making us unable to easily trust those who truly love us and want to care for us. Healthy marital relationships depend on our ability to trust and lower our defenses.

Likewise, the church, the Bride of Christ, can be harmed by relationships with worldly teachers who use the church for selfish means. Private jets and mansions and worldly fame should never be the goal of our spiritual leaders. Their harmful teachings may leave us cynical and guarded, making it hard for us to trust godly leaders who want to lead us to a true, deep relationship with Christ.

If we spend too much time with harmful teachings, we may be left 'infected' with ideas that flare up from time to time, marring our appearance, or worse, that reduce our ability to recognize truth, reducing our 'immunity' to false teaching, eventually leading to poor spiritual health or even spiritual death. Although physically HIV is spread by blood and body fluids and has no cure, our spiritual lives can be cured by the blood of Jesus and the baptism by the Holy Spirit, and the Living Water.

Thankfully, most churches (I believe) have godly leaders who teach truth. Throughout our spiritual lives, we are equipped time after time to share with our lost family, friends, and coworkers. Despite this equipping, we find it hard to do. Many of us live in a spiritual bubble, surrounding ourselves with other Christians so we do not recognize the opportunities when they arise.

Confusion

In recent years, sexual confusion is on the rise. The LGBT movement (with other letters being added over time) has become a powerful force in society. The idea of gender dysphoria, where our genetic code and body type should not define our desired sexual identity, was unheard of through millennia of history, but now has a foothold at least in America. The entertainment industry and social media take great pains to avoid any hint of criticism of those individuals who can ignore biology and pave their own path in society. Even the medical profession has developed specialists who will override our natural bodily systems with hormones and carve our physical bodies to remove unwanted parts or add others to give the appearance we want others to see.

In the Body of Christ, I am not aware of us yet sinking to the depths of confusion noted (although I would not be surprised if there were some who went to extremes analogous to those mentioned above). However, I fear many in the church have limited their social interactions to only those who share the same spiritual body type. These 'homospirituals' rarely interact with unsaved people, or even those of other denominations. Instead, they direct their spiritual affection to fellow Christians and show little compassion to those who are not of the same body.

Some in the LGBT community have a reputation, whether deserved or not, of being quick to protest any disagreement with what they value. Consider the uproar over the Chick-fil-A support of same sex marriage years ago. This became news somewhere around 2010. Even today, we still hear of repercussions related to that stance, although it seems there was no overt opposition to

LGBT causes, but rather support of what we in the church consider traditional marriage.

I believe some in the church have taken a similar approach, giving vocal disagreement against this community. If we are isolated in our affections and limited in our love for others, this can escalate the divide rather than attracting others to the hope of salvation.

Perhaps instead of seeing through that lens, we should consider that all of us, in the church or outside, are "LBGT" (Loved By God Totally). We don't have to agree with other lifestyles to still display God's love.

Summary

The topic of physical reproduction affects each person differently. To some, it is a source of embarrassment or shame, while others make it a source of comedy routines. Some approach it with timidity, others aggressively. Some consider it a right, others a God given act with sacred overtones. With age, many people experience a decrease in their desire to participate in such activities.

In the Body of Christ, reproduction involves making disciples, evangelizing the unchurched, and witnessing to others. In this context, also, some feel embarrassment, some are timid, some are aggressive. As Paul said in 1 Corinthians 9:22: "I have become all things to all men, that I might by all means save some." It is incredible to me that God uses each form of witnessing to reach others. Even the impersonal and sometimes aggressive message of street preachers, when anointed by God, has been known to penetrate the defenses of those prepared by the Spirit and bring conviction, leading them to repentance and salvation.

Older church members may use their age and longevity to withdraw from these activities. For those of us who have lost our 'spiritual libido' or desire to make disciples, the Holy Spirit can transform us, reawakening the desire to share. This cannot and should not be forced on people whom He has not prepared to receive it, but He will put us in situations with people who are receptive to His word. At those 'divine appointments,' our task is to 'Always be ready to give a defense to everyone who asks' (1 Peter 3:15). He will create the opportunities and supply the words needed.

A wise teacher once told me, 'Witness is not something you do; it is something you are.' Our task is to live our lives surrendered to God, seeking Him first. And we must remember, it is not our words or actions that save others, but God, working through us in the hearts of those with whom we interact.

What's in a name

Our patient this time, Inda Metrium, refers to the endometrium. This is the inner lining of the uterus, which thickens and then is shed each month as it prepares to accept a fertilized egg. This physical representation of 1 Peter 3:15 ("Always be ready…") eventually ends at menopause, but spiritually our readiness should continue until our dying breath.

F. The Clinic: Language

Among our peers, and on the chart, doctors use terms and abbreviations that are foreign to our patients. I recall in medical school learning to document notes on a patient's chart. It was like learning a foreign language. Sample documentation of a patient exam would appear like this:

Gen: WDWNWM in NAD, A&O x 3
HEENT: PERLA, TMs wnl
Lungs: CTA
Heart: RRR w/o M
Abd: Soft, NT, no HSM
Neuro: CN II-XII intact

Imagine a new medical student fresh out of college looking at this. To the uninitiated, it is gibberish, and yet now, it makes perfect sense. Translation?

General: Well-developed, well-nourished white male in no acute distress. Alert and oriented x 3 (to person, place, and time)
Head, Eyes, Ears, Nose, and Throat: Pupils equal and reactive to light and accommodation. Tympanic membranes (eardrums) within normal limits
Lungs: Clear to auscultation (i.e., listening with a stethoscope)
Heart: regular rate and rhythm without murmur
Abdomen: soft, non-tender, no hepatosplenomegaly (liver or spleen enlargement)
Neurological: Cranial nerves two through twelve intact. (Cranial nerve one is the olfactory nerve, and seldom would a non-neurologist need to test smell in the exam room, so we skip that one)

In this day of electronic medical records, the alphabet soup of acronyms and abbreviations that we learned in medical school is becoming less common. The computer systems that help us document our exam findings also clean up the shorthand, reducing any confusion it may cause.

In addition, there are legitimate medical terms that have a specific definition that sound harsh to the layman. Popular culture has ruined a few terms for common use, but they are still used on charts. These include mental retardation (yes, that is still a recognized diagnosis, not an insult). Obese refers to an increased body mass index greater than thirty. Spastic describes someone's gait or movements being less smooth because of muscular spasms. And we commonly abbreviate 'shortness of breath' as SOB. If a patient were to read our description of him as obese, with a spastic gait and being SOB, he would understandably be offended despite our completely innocent intentions.

Similarly, people who have not been acclimated to church culture hear us talk about being 'born again.' 'Grace' may be a foreign concept. The term 'covered by the blood' sounds more like a horror movie description outside the church. The early church was accused of practicing cannibalism when people heard them talking about the Lord's supper and partaking of the body and blood of Jesus. There may be confusion about us talking about the lamb and the lion as though they are the same thing (Person?). And demons? Are you serious?

Some terms sound judgmental to the world but we embrace them within our church culture. We are 'sinners,' 'lost,' 'wretched, pitiful, poor, blind and naked' (Rev 3:17). We consider 'surrender' to be a good thing and refer to ourselves as 'servants' or 'slaves' of Christ when our society condemns any reference that honors slavery. The unchurched may hear these as harsh accusations toward those outside the church, not realizing this applies to all of us who are grateful to our savior.

There are societal issues today that play a part as well. I confess I sometimes feel uncomfortable singing some of the popular worship songs. It feels odd to me as a heterosexual adult male to sing songs referring to Jesus as 'precious' or 'beautiful,' but once I get beyond myself, it is perfectly true. To consider myself as part of the Bride of Christ is odd. To someone hearing these references for the first time, I suspect this could be strange.

With more religious education, we hear terms like the canon of scripture, and atonement, propitiation, justification, and sanctification. Even tithe. We refer to people as apologists, evangelists, deacons, or elders. These terms probably mean nothing to someone who has not been steeped in 'church-ese.' And few of us understand how the Trinity looks and functions until we have pondered it for years (even then, our understanding is limited).

Even mature Christians may find some things we talk or sing about awkward. I know some who have struggled with self-confidence would find the words of Amazing Grace uncomfortable, singing that His amazing grace "saved a wretch like me." Or the old hymn '*Alas! and Did My Savior Bleed*' by Isaac Watts in 1707, asking "Would He devote that sacred head for such a worm as I?" Some have referred to this as 'Worm Theology.' A less harsh form of this would be the response popularized by a Christian financial expert, who, when asked 'How are you?" responds that he is "Better than I deserve." Although this is true of us all, some people struggle with understanding the concept of self in comparison to God's grace.

Language is important, but our tone is even more important. Certain topics bring strong emotions. Telling someone they are pregnant should bring joy, but that is not always the case. A diagnosis of cancer is hard to deliver as well as hard to hear. And addressing unhealthy habits such as weight, sexual behaviors, drug use, and other topics can sound judgmental, regardless of how we bring it up.

Likewise, in the church, addressing spiritual health with an accusatory tone or being condescending to those unfamiliar with our language does not draw them to Christ. Without love, we are like a third-grade orchestra concert—out of tune and grating to the ear. Paul described it in 1 Corinthians 13:1, as like a "sounding brass or clanging cymbal."

In my office, I need to use more commonly understood terms to explain things, depending on the level of understanding of my patients. In the church, we need clarity as well. This may involve one-on-one discipleship where we can more clearly convey the wonder of the gospel once we know where the other person's understanding begins. Regardless of the words we use, we must follow the guidance of Paul in Ephesians 4. After talking about God equipping some to be pastors and teachers, strengthening and edifying the Body of Christ, he tells us in verse 15 this needs to be by "speaking the truth in love," so those in the body "may grow up in all things into Him who is the head—Christ."

7

Respiratory—Spirit

> Romans 8:10-11: "But if Christ is in you, then even though your body is subject to death because of sin, the Spirit gives life because of righteousness. And if the Spirit of him who raised Jesus from the dead is living in you, he who raised Christ from the dead will also give life to your mortal bodies because of his Spirit who lives in you." (NIV)

Alvin Oless is 67. He presents to the office with a bad cough and fever. He was eating lunch two days ago and choked. After a few minutes, he was breathing easier but had pain in his chest with each breath. Since then, he has developed chest congestion and a productive cough. He is wheezing and feels out of breath with activity. He developed a fever to 102 degrees yesterday and is concerned about pneumonia. His past medical history is unremarkable, but he smoked cigarettes until he was 48. He takes no daily medications. Other than Tylenol, he has not taken any other medications for his current symptoms. Examination reveals a normal blood pressure, but heart rate is increased to 110, and respiratory rate 20. Temperature is 100 degrees despite taking Tylenol two hours ago. His oxygen saturation is 88% on room air. I hear coarse breath sounds at the base of his right lung. With his low oxygen level and cough, I suspect his choking caused aspiration of food into his lungs leading to aspiration pneumonia. I send him to the hospital to be admitted for IV antibiotics, oxygen, and a chest X-ray.

*****

Our lungs are incredible. They are light and delicate sponges when healthy. As the diaphragm muscle contracts, expanding the chest cavity, the lungs fill with air. The air travels through the main airway called the trachea and branches into smaller and smaller airways—first the bronchi, then the bronchioles, and eventually ending its journey at the small air sacs called alveoli. Each alveolus is fragile, like a bubble, surrounded by tiny blood vessels called capillaries. The exceedingly thin wall of the alveolus, in contact with the thin wall of the capillary, allows oxygen molecules to diffuse across the membranes and bind to the hemoglobin molecules of the red blood cells. Our muscular heart then pumps the oxygenated blood throughout the body, delivering it to each tissue, providing fuel for its designated purpose. The depleted hemoglobin molecules then return to the lungs for a fresh load of oxygen. At each stage of the oxygenation process, problems can occur that interfere with the absorption or delivery of oxygen.

In the Body of Christ, the Holy Spirit is like the air we breathe. Just as oxygen provides fuel to our physical body, He provides power for our spiritual life. The Bible instructs us to live in the Spirit and also walk in the Spirit (Gal 5:25). Anything that hinders our access to the Spirit (i.e., ‘quenches’ the Spirit) can weaken us spiritually.

Absence

Many things can cause trouble with our oxygen levels. The first consideration is simply the absence of oxygen. If we find ourselves in an environment with limited or no air, our lives are in danger. Whether we are trapped in a bank vault or cave, or underwater, or even in outer space, our air supply can be depleted quickly. Without a fresh supply of oxygen, we can quickly lose consciousness or worse.

From a spiritual standpoint, this is not a problem. God's word promises He is always with us. In Psalm 139:7-8 David asks the rhetorical question, "Where can I go from Your Spirit? Or where can I flee from Your presence?" and with each of his examples, his answer is 'You are there.' The Lord Jesus Himself promised "Lo, I am with you always" (Matthew 28:20), and in Deuteronomy 31:6 we are told "the Lord your God, He is the One who goes with you. He will not leave you nor forsake you.." God's omnipresence assures us of His powerful availability at all times.

Despite this assurance, we sometimes limit our access to His presence.

Competition

Exposure to certain chemicals can block our ability to use the oxygen all around us. A common example is carbon monoxide. If we inhale this colorless and odorless gas, it will selfishly bind to the hemoglobin molecule in our red blood cells more quickly and securely than oxygen (one source quotes a 200 times stronger affinity than oxygen. See Toxicological Profile for Carbon Monoxide (cdc.gov)). In this circumstance, even if oxygen is inhaled and absorbed into the bloodstream, it cannot bind to the hemoglobin molecule that is already occupied.

Similarly, worldly affections may attach to our souls, taking our attention. If our priorities shift, we can drift away from the close relationship we once had with God. As we spend time feeding those desires and interests, they may become strong habits or addictions, causing our spiritual health to suffer. Once these take hold in our lives, they may lead to a lifelong struggle of remission and relapse.

Other inhaled gases may reduce oxygen levels in our physical body as well. Nitrous oxide (also known as laughing gas) has had a role in anesthesia for many years. Although it may not have the binding affinity that carbon monoxide does, if it is inhaled in excess concentrations, the reduced amount of oxygen will cause the same end result of hypoxia, or lack of oxygen.

In the spiritual realm, some activities or interests may not rise to the level of addiction. However, if we preferentially surround ourselves with them to the extent that they occupy too much of our time and energy, our attention to spiritual disciplines is reduced, with a similar result of poor spiritual health and lack of strength. In my church, the worship leaders often lead us to practice holding our hands in front of us and opening them as a symbol of releasing burdens and distractions to strengthen our focus on God.

Damage

The fragile tissue of the lungs may be damaged in many ways. For many years, the most common cause of lung disease has been smoking. Decades ago, smoking was so acceptable that cigarettes were advertised in the medical journals, with endorsement by doctors. Cigarettes were commonly provided to soldiers overseas. Nicotine addiction is one of the most difficult to overcome. With ongoing inhalation of toxins in tobacco smoke, damage accumulates in the small, fragile alveoli of the lungs. As these small 'bubbles' break down and join together, they lead to emphysema, forming large bullae that have smaller areas of contact with the capillary system, limiting the diffusion of oxygen into the bloodstream as well as trapping air in the lungs.

A repeated cycle of damage and repair to cells in the body allows the development of mutations leading to cancer. This can cause more extensive destruction as tumors grow, displacing and distorting normal tissue.

Some types of trauma may cause the small alveoli to rupture, allowing air to escape into the tissue surrounding the lung. This 'collapsed lung,' known as a pneumothorax, creates pressure on the wall of the lung, keeping it from properly expanding, not allowing the air to be drawn into the lungs. In some cases, air may be drawn into the pleural space around the lung and become trapped there, blowing up like a balloon and compressing the normal lungs. This is known as a tension pneumothorax.

Spiritually, there may be things that hurt us, keeping us from accepting the truth of God's word. This may lead us to resist God's work in our lives, leading to weakness or struggles spiritually. We may have contact with Spirit-filled teachers and fellowship, but in ourselves be desensitized by past abuses or sins. This is similar to smoking, which causes scarring and damage to our previously healthy lungs. Or there may be some churches where the Bible is not properly taught, but instead, toxic 'cultish' doctrines may lead to damage. I think of the church led by the late Fred Phelps, in Topeka, Kansas, that spent so much energy protesting at funerals and other gatherings. His own children eventually left the church. The danger in that circumstance may be a revulsion toward spiritual truths. This spiritual emphysema may prevent the absorption of truth even if they are exposed to it.

Blockage

Anything that blocks the passage of air into our lungs can cause danger to our physical lives. For example, choking on food or foreign objects acts like a cork, keeping air from entering the lungs. Or an infection such as pneumonia, may cause secretions and bacteria to fill some of the alveoli, leading to swelling of these fragile tissues. Too much mucus, in turn, can plug the bronchioles, keeping air from passing into the smaller tissues.

A common condition for many is asthma. This is a hypersensitivity of the airways that can lead to spasm, squeezing the small airways closed, and increasing mucus production. This can severely limit the flow of air, causing wheezing and shortness of breath. Even in this age of modern medicine, asthma can still be deadly.

Spiritually, there may be circumstances that obstruct our sensitivity to the Holy Spirit. Just as physical obstruction of our airways requires emergency treatment, things that block the work of the Holy Spirit in our lives need urgent attention. False teaching, or interpersonal conflict that stops our spiritual progress causes harm. Certain irritants in our lives may lead to 'spiritual asthma,' causing tension or spasms in our spiritual lives that make us resistant to the work of the Spirit. Left untreated, a physical asthma attack can be deadly, and we need to use a 'rescue inhaler' to relax the airway spasms and allow air to enter our lungs. Spiritually, God is our rescue. We must surrender to him and his work, leading us to being more open to the work of the Spirit.

For an asthma attack, quick use of the rescue inhaler usually provides prompt relief. At times, however, this is not enough. If the airways are inflamed or in spasm, the medicine provided by a quick puff from an inhaler may not penetrate deep enough into the lungs. In such situations, a breathing treatment is used. Using a nebulizer to create a mist that includes the lifesaving medicine, the patient breathes in this medicine for a few minutes, allowing the airways to relax and the lungs to improve. This prolonged exposure to the medicine can have lasting effects.

During a recent church service, while singing and worshipping God, I realized that worship is like a breathing treatment. We are submerged in the Spirit, breathing in His presence, and our souls catch their breath. Deeply breathing in the presence of God can sustain us in the low times, when we are exposed to irritants that could cause us to lose our spiritual breath. In steady doses, He changes our lives.

The Bottom Line

No matter the issue, physically, the result is a lack of absorbing oxygen or circulating it to the tissues of the body. With each problem, the most important thing is to increase our oxygen level. Physically, we add external oxygen, so instead of the natural 21% oxygen in the air, we may need even up to 100% oxygen for short periods of time. This keeps oxygen going to the tissues while we reverse the underlying problem. In cases of more severe illness, mechanical ventilation may be required, using a machine to pump oxygen through an endotracheal tube inserted into the airway instead of depending on a weakened body to draw air in through damaged airways.

Spiritually, impeding the work of the Holy Spirit can be the result of various problems within the Body of Christ. Although many physical respiratory problems cause irreversible damage and chronic problems or even death, spiritual problems are never irreversible if we allow the Spirit to work in our lives. Spending more time in the presence of the Holy Spirit can allow Him to permeate our beings. If there is sin or unhealthy behavior that needs to be corrected, the Lord will prompt us to address that. Once again, surrendering ourselves to God allows Him to do His work in us.

If we are in a church that does not provide proper Bible based teaching, it is as if we physically are in an air-tight box. We may be ok for a short time with the limited amount of oxygen in the box, but as we continue breathing, we exhaust that supply. Without fresh air, we suffocate. Similarly, in a church without fresh Spirit-filled leading and teaching, we weaken spiritually.

Summary

In our physical body, oxygen is vital to life. Each cell in our body depends on a fresh supply of oxygen to metabolize nutrients and maintain function. Every day, as we go about our usual activities, we breathe in new oxygen, usually without even being consciously aware of the process. We can't depend on yesterday's oxygen to support today's life.

Similarly, the Body of Christ requires the presence and work of the Holy Spirit. Without Him, function is futile, and the Body will die. The Spirit provides power and direction, cultivating in us His fruit of love, joy, peace, longsuffering, gentleness, goodness, faith, meekness, and self-control (as listed in Galatians 5:22-23). Our spiritual lives should include daily dependence on Him. We cannot count on past spiritual growth to sustain us for long.

As we walk with God, we should have a constant infilling of the Holy Spirit, praying without ceasing. It should be as natural to us as breathing. Some have noted a similarity to our breathing and to the name of God. As we inhale, we whisper 'Yah' and with each exhalation we whisper 'Weh.' Every moment of the day, God's name, Yahweh, is on our lips if we will but pay attention.

Although many physical respiratory problems cause irreversible damage and chronic problems or even death, thanks be to God that spiritual problems are never irreversible if we allow the Spirit to work in our lives. The Latin word for breathing is what gives us the word inspiration. As we inspire air into our lungs to live, the Spirit inspires us daily to grow in our spiritual life.

What's in a name?

Our patient, Alvin Oless, refers to the alveolus. This is the smallest portion of our lungs, the tiny bubble-like structures where oxygen diffuses across the tissue into the bloodstream for delivery throughout our body. As described above, these fragile tissues are susceptible to damage by inhaled toxins or infections. With accumulated damage, we lose more alveoli, thereby reducing the area of interface between the lungs and the bloodstream and limiting our blood oxygen level.

G. The Clinic: Specialists and Knowledge Base

As a family practitioner, I recognize that my abilities have more breadth than depth. I have limited knowledge of a wide range of conditions, but I sometimes identify a medical problem that my limited abilities are insufficient to treat. At that point, I order a referral to a specialist in that field.

As we go through training, each doctor receives a broad education. During clinical rotations in medical school, we are exposed to various specialties, and many students may then choose to pursue further education in a particular field. They go on to a residency program more focused on their chosen specialty. Some, even beyond residency, will choose to do a fellowship for more specialized and focused training. They then can be certified by the appropriate boards as a specialist, be it in cardiology, nephrology, endocrinology, gastroenterology, or any of the myriad other '-ology's that are available.

Even within the clinic, we have a division of labor. The receptionists have a specific role to play, as do the nurses, the lab techs, the mid-level providers, and the physicians. In small doctor's offices with one provider, he or she and the office nurse may divide all of the jobs, such as checking in patients, taking vital signs, and drawing blood. Larger offices are likely to have more employees taking over certain roles in patient care.

Occasionally, a patient wants me to recheck their blood pressure if it was high when the nurse checked it. This always catches me off guard. I must confess, I feel uncomfortable and awkward doing this simple task since I do it so infrequently. My nurses do this multiple times per day. Although I know how to check it, I am not as practiced and efficient at it as my nurse.

Similarly, the church has a similar range of duties. In a small church, the pastor may do the preaching and hospital visits, while volunteers (or his own family members) help with administrative duties, youth programs, and music. As the church grows, more work is involved in each aspect of ministry, and subsequently, the staff will likely grow. On a particular church staff, there may be a senior pastor, an executive or associate pastor, a youth pastor, a minister of music, a children's pastor, and sometimes others. The larger the church, the larger the staff is likely to be.

This division of labor allows more direct ministry to the needs of each group. Although the senior pastor is able to minister to the youth in the church, a full-time youth pastor can devote more time to addressing the specific culture and interests of that age group. Typically, being of a younger age than the senior pastor assists him or her in engaging the youth and discipling them for a closer walk with Christ. Similarly, a music minister can devote more time to organizing a choir or worship team. Although talent should not supersede someone's walk with Christ, a more practiced team of musicians may help the congregation worship more than a kind, less talented volunteer whose performance overshadows the message of the song.

Medically, it seems new information is published every year. New testing, screening recommendations, classes of medications, and surgical techniques seem to be the norm. And of course, our recommended schedule of vaccinations has become much more crowded.

In my practice, I tend to stick with tried-and-true methods of treatment. The new things advertised to the public may be new and improved, but that usually comes with a price tag and may not be covered by insurance. Just because it is new and improved does not mean prior methods no longer work.

Unfortunately, there are also new discoveries that contradict former practices. Just a few examples since I started practice more than thirty years ago include cholesterol treatment guidelines, use of aspirin in primary prevention of heart disease, use of anesthesia for circumcision, cervical cancer screening guidelines, hormone replacement after menopause, and use of opioids in treating chronic pain. Even some ancient practices were abandoned, and are now in use again. For example, leeches were a mainstay of treatment centuries ago, then viewed as barbaric. Now, some aspects of care still find them useful.

When the treatment fails, or if the patient presents with something beyond my abilities, I have the option of referring to someone specialized in that condition. Those who are specialists have spent years treating a specific body system or disease process. They are practiced in treatments that are more effective when common ones fail. Their knowledge has been honed by their focus and emphasis on that particular problem area.

In the Body of Christ, there are many training programs for specialty staff positions. Learning what has or has not worked in certain areas of ministry can save time and expense by avoiding mistakes. Sharing educational or ministry materials can enhance ministry as well.

As time progresses, styles of ministry change, as do the cultural needs of each group. This division of labor allows each minister to enhance his ability to relate to those under his care within the church.

As we have noted, the physical body may not have changed much through the years, but our approach to caring for it sure has. It is a constant battle to keep up to date with new treatments. Shelves are filled with thick, expensive books on each specialty.

From a spiritual standpoint, we have one 'textbook' on which we rely. Through the years, there have been competing interpretations of the Bible, but the basic orthodox doctrines have remained consistent. The fact remains that Jesus died to pay the price for our sins and offers His gift of eternal life to any who will open the door to him. We don't need to be specialized in our training for that to happen.

8

Cardiovascular—Distribution

Romans 10:14-15 (NIV) "How, then, can they call on the one they have not believed in? And how can they believe in the one of whom they have not heard? And how can they hear without someone preaching to them? And how can anyone preach unless they are sent?"

Cordell Tindenny, age 53, comes in because his heart is racing. For the past few weeks, he has had episodes of rapid heartbeat that take his breath away and cause him to feel dizzy. These episodes last five to ten minutes and are becoming more frequent, now occurring daily. There is no identifiable trigger, and the episodes are not related to exertion. His medical history includes hypothyroidism, and he has not come in for lab work for two years. He takes his wife's leftover thyroid medicine, but the dose is higher than what was prescribed for him.

His examination indicates his blood pressure is 134/82, and heart rate 84 beats per minute, or bpm. His body mass index is 27, and his weight is six kilograms lower than it was when we last saw him a year ago. As we are talking, he experiences another episode. His heart is now tachycardic with a rate of approximately 140 bpm. I ask for an electrocardiogram (also known as an EKG), which shows supraventricular tachycardia, documenting his rate at 162 bpm. As we talk about the findings and prepare to send him to the emergency room, his symptoms resolve, and re-examination shows his heart rate back to 96. Repeat EKG now shows sinus rhythm and a rate of 94.

Laboratory work confirms that his thyroid is overactive on the borrowed pills. I lower his dose and refer him to cardiology, but I expect his rhythm will remain normal.

*****

The cardiovascular system is amazing. Every day, our heart functions without our conscious thought to pump blood, first to the lungs to collect oxygen and then again to every organ in our body to supply the nutrients, minerals, and oxygen required for each one to function. The blood travels through the strong-walled arteries as they steadily narrow in each organ, and then returns via the system of ever-enlarging veins back to the heart for another trip. Along the way, the blood passes through the kidney, liver, and spleen to be analyzed and cleansed of toxins and broken or outdated cells. Our heart pumps an average of sixty to one hundred twenty beats every minute, every day of our lives. This is automatically adjusted for activity, stress, illness, and injury.

The heart is actually two pumps in one. The right side of the heart collects blood returning from its journey through the body, now depleted of oxygen. As the right ventricle contracts, it pumps blood through the pulmonary arteries in a short trip to the lungs to collect a fresh supply of oxygen. (One bit of medical trivia: the pulmonary arteries are the only *arteries* in the body that carry *unoxygenated* blood, and pulmonary *veins* are similarly unique as they return *oxygenated* blood to the heart.) As the blood returns from the lungs to the left side of the heart, it is pumped by the larger left ventricle out to the body for a longer trip.

As we follow unhealthy lifestyles, our weight increases, causing the muscular heart to work harder, and like other muscles in the body, as its workload increases, the heart enlarges. The muscular walls of the arteries will thicken or 'harden' as well. High levels of fat in our diet, aided by genetic factors, can cause plaque to accumulate inside our arteries like corrosion in our pipes at home. Eventually, the plaque may rupture and block the arteries that feed the heart muscle itself, causing part of the heart to be starved of oxygen, leading to an infarction, where some of the heart muscle cells die. Depending on the amount of heart muscle affected, this 'heart attack' has the potential to greatly weaken or even stop the heart completely, leading to death.

Aside from the circulatory system that supplies the heart muscle, it also has a sophisticated electrical system. This naturally designed pacemaker sends an electrical signal for each heartbeat. The signal starts in the upper chambers of the heart at the sinus node and then is transmitted down the 'wires' called bundle branches to each side of the heart. If it follows its design properly, this divided signal reaches each lower chamber simultaneously, causing these larger ventricles to contract and pump the blood efficiently.

This electrical system of the heart can be disrupted in many ways, causing an irregular rhythm. If the rhythm is not regulated, the upper chambers of the heart may not properly pump to fill the lower chambers. The lower chambers may then beat irregularly, sending out a smaller volume of blood with each contraction. Or, as in the case of our patient noted above, the pacemaker may fire too rapidly. Even though the rhythm is regular, it is so fast it does not allow time for blood to fill the heart, so it, again, pumps inefficiently and a smaller volume of blood is dispersed each time.

The four valves in the heart function to direct flow in the proper direction. As the upper chambers of the heart contract, they pump blood to the lower chamber through one-way valves that are pushed open by the force of blood being pumped, and then the leaflets of the valves slam shut to prevent backflow. It is the slamming of the valves that causes the familiar and soothing 'lub dub' of our heart sounds, the 'lub' caused by the valves between the atria and ventricles closing (tricuspid valve on the right side and mitral valve on the left). Then the larger, more muscular part of the heart pumps the blood forcefully out of the heart through another pair of valves. On the right side, the pulmonic valves prevent backflow to the right ventricle, and on the left, the aortic valve. The closing of this second set of valves provides the 'dub' of our heart sounds.

If any of the valves do not function properly, a practiced ear can hear the 'swoosh' of blood instead of the decisive lub or dub. This may occur with narrowing of the valves restricting flow and causing a traffic jam of blood, like putting your thumb over a garden hose to spray it. Conversely, the valves can malfunction and not close properly, allowing blood to regurgitate backwards, leading to back pressure and less efficient flow of blood.

This is, of course, a simplified look at the function and problems of the heart. Cardiologists who specialize in treating problems of circulation are kept extremely busy with these issues and many other conditions that arise. Their specialty is even subdivided into those that treat electrical problems by doing specialized procedures, those that open blocked arteries with stents, those that fix problematic valves, and those that treat general concerns of the heart, such as blood pressure and cholesterol.

Obviously, our physical cardiovascular system is incredibly important to our overall health. And, of course, there are parallels in the spiritual body.

As we read the Bible, God refers to the heart many times. Generally, the scriptural reference to the heart has to do with the inner being, thoughts, emotions, and character. For the purposes of this chapter, however, I plan to focus more on the practical aspects of the physical heart and how they have parallels in the spiritual body, the church. More properly, we are dealing with the circulatory system.

Distribution

I consider physical circulation to be akin to the distribution of the Gospel message and spiritual truth. A clear message of spiritual truth is sent out in the form of a sermon, worship song, book, podcast, or other media. It reaches those who are spiritually hungry or needing renewal, bringing what is needed for spiritual health.

In the early days of the church, our Lord started with the disciples and face-to-face, word-of-mouth evangelism. This is still the way humanity is saved, one soul at a time, personally hearing the Gospel message and responding. However, as with most things, mankind takes good, simple things and tries to improve them. Through the ensuing millennia, the Body of Christ has developed systems and protocols and agendas to reach more people with the Gospel, and these programs and methods require support and structure to keep them functioning. And yet God still works. People hear the message, read the word, respond to the prompting of the Holy Spirit, and His Kingdom comes, and His will is done on earth as it is in heaven. The modern church can be very effective in reaching the lost around the world if we continue to humbly seek God's will and direction.

Vessels

As our heart pumps, it sends out life-giving blood throughout the body. This carries oxygen and nutrients to each organ, maintaining function and health. This requires a system of arteries and veins, as well as the muscle action of the heart's pump and the electrical activity of the heart's rhythm.

I envision this as strong, healthy churches sending out missionaries or church planters to far-reaching areas of the world. As they are 'pumped out' into the world, these servants carry the milk and meat of the Word of God, facilitating the 'oxygen' of the Holy Spirit's work in the lives of unreached people.

The sending of missionaries is accomplished through various systems, such as mission organizations, denominations that support their own missionaries with church budgets, and local churches that support individual missionaries or church planters. The more complex the systems become, the more opportunities for breakdown to occur. This can limit the supply of money or supplies needed for the missionaries to function. Most vital is prayer support.

Regardless of human systems, God can and will reach people in ways that we cannot even imagine. The work of the Holy Spirit is not dependent on missionaries, and there are ongoing reports of people, especially in Muslim countries, having visions of Jesus leading them to seek Him.

Stents

We all know that 2020 was a terrible year in society around the world. The pandemic brought many aspects of life to a halt. In-person church services, like most group gatherings, ceased to exist for several months. Just like a heart attack causing severe limits to our physical circulation and threatening our physical health, we suffered limits and challenges that had the potential to threaten our spiritual health. But Jesus promised that the gates of hell would not prevail against His Church.

Many churches changed to virtual worship. I liken this to a stent for our heart. This is a small tubular brace that is inserted in the blocked artery and expanded, holding it open and restoring patency. This restores circulation that has stopped and allows function to continue. Our physical hearts may never be fully restored to normal if there has been damage to the heart muscle, but spiritually, God is not limited. As we come back together in corporate worship, there may be some changes that are ongoing, but we are once again the Church Body together.

Arrhythmia

Physically, there can be arrhythmias causing the heartbeat to be erratic and unreliable. This inefficiency of cardiac output can frequently cause weakness, dizziness, breathlessness, and physical limitations.

Spiritually, the Body of Christ may suffer inefficiencies in many ways. It may be infrastructure that limits access in third-world countries, or political restrictions in some countries that outlaw Christianity and any form of evangelism, or even owning a Bible. There are still many countries and people groups around the world that do not have printed Bibles in their own language, limiting direct access to God's written word.

Closer to home, we may see poor function in the form of sermons targeted at social issues instead of God's word, or unorthodox teachings, legalistic requirements or worship choruses that have spiritually confusing messages or untruths. Bookstores are full of spiritual and 'Christian' books that may contradict each other and put forward a particular agenda, rather than Biblical truth. It takes discernment and spiritual wisdom as we consider what we hear, testing it in the light of God's word.

Congestive heart failure

Physically, we may suffer from congestive heart failure when the heart is weakened. Instead of pumping the blood volume forward, the inefficiency causes a 'back up' that can cause swelling in our legs, as well as fluid in our lungs. As this occurs, we are unable to comfortably lie flat to sleep, and we become short of breath when we do any activity. The heart is then grossly enlarged and 'flabby,' pumping a smaller volume of blood with each beat, limiting the delivery of blood to our organs.

Spiritually, we sometimes see bloated megachurches that seem to have swollen attendance numbers, and occasionally this leads to weakened spiritual messages designed to avoid alienating the congregation rather than to equip them for service. Thankfully, this is not common, and even the largest churches can have a tremendous impact on reaching the unchurched with the good news of the Gospel.

Valvular disease

As described earlier, our heart valves may at times become diseased. This can be a result of infection, autoimmune problems, physical damage, and heart attacks, to name just a few causes. The valves can become narrowed or leaky, and both problems can be dangerous. Physically, valves can be replaced to reapproximate normal function.

Spiritually, a leaky valve may be compared to gossip. We spend our time passing information in the wrong direction, wasting energy and time that prevents forward progress of some members of the Body. Conversely, narrowed valves may be likened to obstinate, stubborn members that spend time and energy opposing or blocking forward progress.

Thankfully, God can and does heal these conditions when we humble ourselves and seek His forgiveness and direction.

Summary

Our circulatory system provides a conduit for delivering necessary oxygen and nutrition to all of our organs. Each step of this process is vital to our health, and any problems along the way can impair us.

Spiritually, we have developed systems to deliver 'nutrition' in the way of teaching all around the world. Without this interconnectedness, people in remote areas would not have the same access to the word of God, or spiritual teaching that is now available in the developed world.

The Great Commission has not expired. Our churches locally and worldwide exist to proclaim the good news of Jesus to those who don't yet know. Yes, we have a lot of structures and programs and systems, but if we hold them loosely, letting God do with them as He wishes, people around the world can be impacted with the truth of God's love for them. Our seminaries provide education and training, and we continue to see new churches being planted and missionaries being sent to parts of the world where Jesus has not yet been proclaimed.

Jesus said, "In the same way your Father in heaven is not willing that any of these little ones should perish." (Matthew 18:14, NIV). We should share the same concern that His name be proclaimed around the world.

What's in a name?

Cordell Tindenny refers to the chordae tendineae. These are fibrous cords that attach to the mitral and aortic valves to keep them from swinging too far into the atria, thus preventing backflow of blood in the wrong direction. Picture a swinging door that needs to be stabilized to only swing in one direction, so a chain is attached to one side to keep it from going too far. In rare cases where these cords rupture, this allows severe valvular regurgitation and generally necessitates surgical correction. Some people refer to these as the heartstrings, but tugging on these heartstrings is not advisable.

H. The Clinic: Assumptions

When you mention having a doctor's appointment, people conjure up certain mental images. The stereotype may be that you wait for an hour, then the doctor only spends a few minutes with you. They bill you excessively and prescribe a bunch of pills that cause a variety of side effects. They want you to have embarrassing or uncomfortable tests. The doctor may be greedy and arrogant, not really caring about you or listening to your concerns. The true facts you found on the internet and brought in to direct your care are ignored. They want you to take vaccines that everybody knows will kill you. And many more. It seems people develop preconceived notions about medicine, and in the age of internet 'enlightenment,' there are more seemingly every day.

The church may trigger similar preconceptions. For example, they are full of hypocrites, they only want your money, they are judgmental. The ones who really believe this stuff are weird. They don't believe in having fun. They try to force their beliefs on everyone. They think they are right and everyone else is wrong. They caused all the wars in history by trying to force their beliefs on others. If they were really Christians, they would give you what you need when you ask. If you joined them, you would have to give up everything you like to do. And their music is so lame!

Medically, patients may downplay their health problems. "It's just indigestion, my cholesterol is not that bad." "My dad was overweight, and he didn't get diabetes until he was older." "My drug and alcohol use are under control." "The doctor is heavier than I am." "My exercise and healthy habits will save me, so I don't need to go to the doctor." "My chiropractor or nutritionist is better than going for a checkup."

People in the world may similarly feel they are not as bad as others around them. "I do nice things for people." "The church family at the next table just complained to the waitress, and I would never do that, so I am better than they are." "I can believe in The Force, or Buddhist philosophy, and meditate a few days a week. That is better than going to church." "My exercise and healthy habits will save me, so who needs church?"

These prejudices may cause patients to delay or avoid getting medical care that can save their lives. Even more tragically, these wrong opinions about the body of Christ can cause many to miss hearing the Good News of salvation.

One day, the indigestion turns into crushing chest pain and shortness of breath, or the drug and alcohol use catch up with them, and they end up in the ER. Then they get medical care for a more serious health issue than before, and realize how much of life they are missing because of failure to seek care sooner.

Or their self-sufficient lifestyle causes a crisis in their life, and the things they enjoy are taken from them. In desperation, they find themselves in a hotel room, and the Gideon Bible shows them the Way of hope and peace. They relent and go to church and realize they had wrong assumptions that caused them to miss out on joy for too many years.

The Word of God says they will know we are Christians by our love (John 13:35). But we somehow need to have contact and interaction with them for them to see that Love in person and in the person of Jesus. We may need to reach out to some skeptical people to overcome their prejudices against us.

Almost all assumptions are based on some level of truth. Yes, there are doctors who are arrogant, condescending, and greedy. Similarly, we are all too familiar with famous preachers who have moral failures or seem to be greedily wanting donations. Our lives need to reflect Jesus, but since we are sinful and fallen human beings, we will never do this perfectly until we reach heaven.

However, as we take up our crosses daily and die to self repeatedly, we will hopefully model the attitude of John the Baptist when he said, "He must increase, but I must decrease." (John 3:30, NKJV). This is commanded in scripture where we are told "but as He who called you is holy, you also be holy in all your conduct, because it is written, 'Be holy, for I am holy.'" (1 Peter 1:6). This is the true meaning of sanctification, becoming holy as we are set apart for His service, and should be a part of all our lives.

9

Nervous System—Getting the Message

Isaiah 30:21 "Your ears shall hear a word behind you, saying, "This is the way, walk in it," whenever you turn to the right hand or whenever you turn to the left."

Otto Nahmyk is 37 and is a computer programmer. He comes in complaining that his right hand has been 'falling asleep' for the past two weeks. He has been spending his evenings and weekends finishing his basement, and this problem with his hand started after he had spent the better part of a weekend using his hammer and screwdriver. When he works on his projects, the right hand develops a tingling 'pins and needles' feeling in most of his fingers and his palm. If he stops working and shakes his hand briefly, this sensation resolves for a while, only to return after he resumes his work. He also has this sensation in the night at times. Since this began, it seems to be happening more frequently, and now he is also noticing it when he types on his keyboard or uses his computer mouse at work.

The history and physical in my office indicate that he has been otherwise healthy and is on no regular medications. He has a normal blood pressure, and the exam is unrevealing, with normal sensation during the office visit and no sign of impairment in using his hand.

I advise him he has carpal tunnel syndrome due to repetitive motion and recommend he wear a wrist support with activity and take a non-steroidal anti-inflammatory medication. It will likely improve as he finishes his project and reduces his activity. If it does not, we will refer him to a hand specialist who can discuss surgical options with him.

*****

Our nervous system is incredibly complex, controlling all of the major functions in our bodies. The master control is our brain, protected by the thick bony armor of the skull. Signals are transmitted from the brain through the nerves traveling down the spinal cord and fanning out to all areas of the body. The brain and nerves are delicate and fragile. The nerves extending from the brain are some of the longest cells in the body, extending several yards from the brain to the farthest reach of the extremities.

Problems of the nervous system are roughly sorted into three categories: Initiation, transmission, or reception. (This is by no means all encompassing, but for the purposes of this book will suffice.)

1. Initiation: By this, I mean just about any problem in the brain. Migraine headaches are a common complaint. Certain tremors or movement disorders begin in the brain, such as Parkinson's disease. An increasingly common diagnosis in recent years is Alzheimer's disease, which affects the brain tissue. The brain can be affected by stroke, tumor,

concussion, infection, parasite, and many other problems. If the nerve impulse is not formed properly, it cannot have the desired effect on the body.

2. Transmission: Once this nerve impulse begins, it needs to be transmitted to the body. Diseases of the peripheral nerves can be localized or widespread. Spinal cord issues, such as disk herniation or injury, can be severely limiting. Nerve compression, such as the carpal tunnel syndrome described in our patient, Otto, may be minor or severe. Cuts on the fingers may damage a cutaneous nerve, which can cause localized numbness distal to the injury. Peripheral neuropathy, whether it be from diabetes or vitamin B12 deficiency or other causes, can lead to chronic burning discomfort of the extremities. These are just a few examples. The nerve impulse may be formed perfectly, but if it can't be sent properly to the rest of the body, the effect is not what it should be.
3. Reception: The third category of nerve-related disorders involves the effect of the nerve impulse when it reaches its destination, specifically in triggering muscle action. One major disease of the neuromuscular junction is myasthenia gravis, but there are other rare causes. Certain toxins or venoms can block this effect as well, such as botulism, snake venom, organophosphates found in some pesticides, and even excess blood levels of magnesium. Injection of botulinum toxin (commonly known as Botox) to specific small areas is a well-known cosmetic treatment for wrinkles, but can also be used in treating vocal cord spasms, migraines, and many other problems. In these conditions, the nerve impulse is formed properly and transmitted well to the muscle, but when it gets there, the muscle cannot respond.

In comparing the physical nervous system to the spiritual body, I am glad to say category one listed above is not a problem. The head of the Body is Christ, and He is perfect, never failing. The 'spiritual nerve impulses' from Him as he leads through the Holy Spirit are given to us in various ways; sometimes directly through prayer and Bible reading, and often through our spiritual leaders—pastors, teachers, and evangelists.

Transmission

Although the message is given by God, if it is not transmitted to us fully and clearly, the spiritual Body will not have the proper impact on the world around us. Maybe a pastor feels led to preach a certain message, but waters it down or does not deliver it fully. Perhaps he is worried about criticism or backlash, or loss of church members.

Just as damage to our physical nerves inhibits function, our leaders and teachers may fall into moral failure that damages their effectiveness. Or, like a pinched nerve physically, the pressures surrounding our leaders may overwhelm them. Stress and anxiety are widespread in church leadership positions, and when it reaches a certain threshold, their abilities may be impaired.

We must continue to pray for our leaders as they spur us on in our relationship with Christ.

Reception

Physically, problems receiving nerve impulses can be attributed to toxins or autoimmune processes. Spiritual toxins are outside influences that poison us or paralyze us. Persecutions or temptations for which we are not prepared can weaken us and paralyze us in our response to God.

Autoimmune problems come from within. Fellow churchgoers who have not surrendered to Christ can influence weaker members, or false doctrines and practices propagated by those who are not trained leaders. Members attacking each other and undermining their service will lead to harm, damaged relationships, and limited function of the body.

Phantom Pain

One other unique problem with nerve signals is Phantom Pain Syndrome. When a patient has required amputation of an extremity, a common complication is the sensation of discomfort or outright pain in the appendage that is no longer present. Some sources say up to 95% of amputees will experience a sensation of discomfort in an amputated extremity. The severity of this can vary, but at times it can be debilitating.

Throughout our lives, the peripheral nerves constantly report back to the central nervous system. These constant status reports give valuable information on position, pain, overuse, heat, cold, and so on. When a nerve is severed, as with an amputation, suddenly, the nerve feedback goes silent. Without this stream of information, sometimes our bodies fill in the emptiness with perceived signals that are not accurate, such as pain in the absent structure. Even though the toe is missing, the patient may feel an uncomfortable itching sensation in a place they can't scratch.

Spiritually, we sometimes misinterpret the words or actions of another person. We may perceive a hurt where none was intended, or attribute wrong motives to someone. In other words, we perceive a signal that was not sent. Anger and bitterness can occur toward someone who is oblivious to our response, since they did nothing to trigger such a response.

Forgiveness can be difficult, but is necessary. Sometimes we must seek forgiveness for our misperceptions since the other party is not at fault. We must learn to give grace, expecting good motives even when our first response is anger. Seeing beyond our emotions takes practice and maturity in our walk with Christ.

The Autonomic Nervous System

Every day, our physical body systems function without our conscious thought. Our heart beats, our eyes blink, we breathe even when we sleep, and our food digests and moves through our gastrointestinal tract. These necessary functions in our body are too important to leave to our conscious control. We are too easily distracted to depend on our will for these vital actions. Imagine if all day long we were reminding ourselves to breathe or to swallow or to blink!

These involuntary functions are under the control of the autonomic nervous system. This division of the nervous system allows our organs to function without our conscious awareness. If a crumb or drop of water gets into our airway, even before we are aware of it, our diaphragm contracts and we cough forcefully to expel this intruder. If we walk out of a dark room into bright sunlight, our pupils automatically constrict, and we squint to limit the amount of light that could cause damage to our delicate retina. If we step on something sharp, our foot automatically withdraws, and we jump away from the painful stimulus. In times of danger, our 'fight or flight' response kicks in, releasing adrenaline to raise our heart rate and prepare us for action.

Considering the Body of Christ, many times we are not aware of what God is up to. We all may have times when we feel spiritually numb or alone, but God is still working. He supplies needs before we realize we are lacking, or sets 'divine appointments' for us to cross paths with someone who needs His touch. He prepares us for action with a new infilling of the Holy Spirit, like divine adrenaline. When something threatens, He many times supplies the reflex actions needed for protection. Even in the dark times, He works to build and uphold His Body, the Church.

Just as our autonomic nervous system works without our input, God's word tells us "…for it is God who works in you both to will and to do for His good pleasure." (Philippians 2:13)

Summary

Our nervous system affects every part of our body, sending messages for either voluntary or involuntary action. The message starts in the brain, travels through the spinal cord, and extends outward through the peripheral nerves to cause action where it is desired.

Spiritually, we also must receive and act on messages sent to us as members of the Body of Christ. Problems may occur with the transmission of His message, but Christ is the head of the body, and He does not fail.

Throughout our lives, God works in us and through us. Just like the autonomic division of the nervous system, God is at work even when we do not perceive it. He accomplishes His will in ways we may never know, and He sustains us during those times of spiritual drought when we may not sense His presence.

When Jesus healed paralytics in the Gospel records, He (the head) delivered a direct message ('nerve impulse') to the afflicted and they received it with dramatic results. May we also, as His Body, receive His message and act with dramatic results.

What's in a name?

Our patient this time is Otto Nahmyk. By now, you realize this refers to the autonomic nervous system, the part of our nervous system that works without relying on our conscious direction. This has far-reaching effects in the body, directing our internal organs, our digestion, our pupil size, blinking, withdrawal from pain, coughing, and so on. If you are a control freak, I'm sorry, but this part of you needs to function without your control!

I. The Clinic: House Calls

For centuries, medicine was mobile. The sick and injured were not required or expected to travel to a medical center, but the physician would go to them. Even a century ago, house calls were still common, and the comfortable TV picture of the kindly old General Practitioner with his doctor's bag visiting a sick patient in their own bedroom as the concerned family gathered around is still what many long for. There are physicians who continue to make house calls, but in an age of limited insurance reimbursement and high overhead expenses, including malpractice insurance, this is diminishing. Now, right or wrong, the usual model is a crowded waiting room, with patients being ushered to an exam room for their turn with the busy doctor. When their fifteen-minute appointment is over, the next patient is brought back. This allows the doctor to more efficiently use his time to see the maximum number of patients.

When a patient is too sick to come to the office, or when they are partially recovered from a hospital but still needing care, it usually falls to the home health nurses and therapists to visit them in their homes, assessing their needs, providing dressing changes for wounds, or injection therapy, or physical therapy.

Clinics and hospitals do, at times, participate in community outreach. It may be a health fair with free blood pressure checks, or a free clinic at a homeless shelter, as a way of reaching out to the people with limited access to healthcare. Medical mission trips or organizations such as Doctors Without Borders take this a step further, reaching out to underserved people in other countries. However, although caring for the sick is a primary tenet of medicine, most of us are content to leave the outreach to a select few while we maintain our routine.

The church today also seems to follow the 'Field of Dreams' strategy: if you build it (i.e., the church building), they will come. The larger the attendance, the greater the status in the community and denomination. This can also provide a larger budget for programs to minister to the congregation.

Of course, at the beginning of the church in Acts, the disciples would go to the people. Paul would enter the local synagogue. Phillip went to the Ethiopian Eunuch. Jesus gave the Great Commission to go into all the world. Throughout church history, there have been circuit preachers who went from town-to-town preaching. Tent revivals were a common outreach tool a century ago. More recently, citywide crusades were commonly held. I well remember as a teenager attending such events. Today, churches around the world make it a priority to reach the people in their local community, and missionaries go to virtually every country to spread the Gospel.

Each of these outreach programs, whether for medicine or for evangelism, are initial steps. They serve to introduce people to medical care they may not have known they needed. Or to bring the Gospel to unchurched people who then become aware of their spiritual needs. At that point, they are directed to an established primary care doctor or specialist for ongoing care, or spiritually to a supportive church where they are discipled in their spiritual walk.

To be honest, I am not offended by the current systems in either medical care or the church. These arrangements, both for medical practices and for churches, facilitate the delivery of care to a larger population than could be reached with either individual house calls or with one-on-one discipleship. But for those with poor understanding or poor access to either medical or spiritual support, we must have a way of reaching out to them, to invite them in, to educate and care for them.

10

Immune system—Remember

Exodus 13:8-10, "And you shall tell your son in that day, saying, 'This is done because of what the Lord did for me when I came up from Egypt.' It shall be as a sign to you on your hand and as a memorial between your eyes, that the Lord's law may be in your mouth; for with a strong hand the lord has brought you out of Egypt. You shall therefore keep the ordinance in its season from year to year."

Anna Flaxus is 26. She comes in to see me for a rash on her face. It has been occurring across her cheeks on both sides at various times. In addition, she has had aching in her joints, which seems to be progressing, and she recently saw blood in her urine. She is on no regular medications and has been in good health up until now.

On examination, her blood pressure is 133/84, and her body mass index is 26. Her lungs are clear, and her heartbeat is regular. She has no pain on palpation of her abdomen. I see a pink rash across her cheeks in a butterfly distribution. I suspect she may have systemic lupus erythematosus and order labs. They return showing a high Anti-Nuclear Antibody level, and her sedimentation rate is increased, reinforcing my suspicions. Her kidney function is mildly reduced, and her urine shows traces of blood. I refer her to a rheumatology specialist.

*****

Immune Response

Our immune system is marvelous. We can be exposed to a particular infection like measles in childhood, and, like a factory in wartime, our bone marrow begins churning out antibodies that are specific to this virus. Once we heal from this disease, the blueprint for this particular antibody is kept on file, with a few antibodies always circulating, on patrol in case there is another invasion. If we are exposed to measles again, our antibodies recognize this familiar foe and signal for reinforcements. If necessary, many more antibodies are produced and join the battle to repel this attack quickly and efficiently, and we may never even realize it occurred. The immune system acts as our memory of infections, allowing us to identify and take control of previously defeated germs early before they spread.

Spiritually, as the Body of Christ, our memory of things we personally experienced acts as our natural immunity. This gives us a vivid memory of the problems resulting from our own sin and wayward behavior, and triggers in us an early response to temptation before it takes root. As we take heed to our conscience, reminding us of the consequences of sin, we can turn away from the path of disobedience.

In our physical bodies, the immune system allows us to resist infections that attack. Spiritually, we are likewise urged to "Resist the devil and he will flee from you." (James 4:7). Our spiritual immunity grows stronger with each act of resistance.

Of course, the same passage of scripture goes on to tell us "Draw near to God and He will draw near to you. Cleanse your hands, you sinners; and purify your hearts, you double-minded." (James 4:8). This serves to remind us of the fact that avoidance of infection or of temptation is safer than exposure. There is always the risk that our immune defenses can be overwhelmed, putting our lives at risk, whether it be physically or spiritually.

Immunizations

Historically, some infections have been devastating to the population. Whether it be smallpox, polio, influenza, or Covid, epidemics have at times brought severe hardship to populations around the world. The World Health Organization, as of this writing, has estimated a cumulative death toll from COVID-19 of 7.1 million people (http://covid19.who.int , accessed 9/28/2025).

With each pandemic threat, medical researchers worked tirelessly to find ways to treat these terrible diseases, but even more to prevent them from taking hold in the first place. As medical knowledge advanced, it was discovered that weakened forms of certain pathogens could be deliberately injected to induce an immune response without causing the actual infection.

In the 1790s, smallpox caused widespread devastation. Edward Jenner, a physician in England, heard stories that milkmaids who had contracted cowpox, a much milder infection which was caused by a virus known as vaccinia (from the Latin word for cow), did not catch smallpox. In May of 1796, he tested this information by inoculating an eight-year-old boy with matter from fresh cowpox lesions. This young patient developed a mild illness for 24 hours and then recovered. Two months later, Jenner took the bold step of inoculating him with actual smallpox from a patient with fresh lesions (a research study that would be condemned today), and he had no smallpox lesions. Thus, vaccinations were born, named after Vaccinia, the viral cause of cowpox.

With the overwhelming evidence of the effectiveness and safety of vaccines, by the 1940's they were recommended for all children. (Vaccine History: Developments by Year | Children's Hospital of Philadelphia (chop.edu)). Initially, this just included smallpox, diphtheria, tetanus, and pertussis. Eventually, the polio epidemic triggered the discovery of the Salk vaccine. Through the years since then, there have been numerous vaccines added, each with proven benefit at saving lives and preventing disease. The effectiveness of vaccination led to the worldwide eradication of smallpox in the 1970s.

Although our immune systems have long memories of these benefits, we as a people do not. As our memories of the devastation from vaccine-preventable diseases faded, a growing minority of people began protesting the recommendations and school requirements, feeling their freedom had been taken away. As social media became a stronger influence, misinformed opinions spread as fact. This was overwhelmingly on display with the recent COVID-19 vaccine. Even as the hospitals filled with a surge of illness among unvaccinated people, there remained a strong resistance and outright distrust of the vaccine.

In the Body of Christ, we hope to keep our members from experiencing the consequences of sin. Like smallpox, some sins can produce lifelong disfiguring scars on our souls. We want to prevent this before it takes root. That is where induced immunity has value. Just like a vaccine benefits us physically, causing us to develop defenses against illnesses we have not personally seen, spiritually we also gain benefit from others in identifying and defending against the wrong path.

The Old Testament is full of accounts that remind the children of Israel of God's deliverance. Frequently, the patriarchs set up stones of remembrance of God's faithfulness. And as noted in the verses at the beginning of this chapter, the annual celebration of the Passover, like a yearly flu shot, was a way to remind the Jewish people of God's deliverance.

It used to be common in smaller churches to have times of testimony, where those in the congregation could stand and share what God was doing in their lives. Accounts of spiritual victories can bring hope and strengthen resolve to fight temptation. In the absence of testimonies of other church members, sermons from the pulpit and reading accounts of heroes of the faith can help shore up our defenses. Accounts of God's miraculous intervention bring hope in the midst of our own struggles, boosting our faith. We need constant reminders because we have short memories.

Passive immunity

Newborns, for the most part, have a blank slate when it comes to their immune system. They have not yet been exposed to pathogens that are common and widespread in our daily lives. If they are attacked by germs like the common cold virus, they are not equipped to defend themselves. Thankfully, God designed us in such a way that babies in the womb inherit short-term immunity from their mothers. Both through shared blood supply in the womb and through breast milk when nursing, immunoglobulins are available that protect them at their most vulnerable stage of life. This immunity is passive, taking no effort on the part of the patient but using the experienced immune system of the mother.

Another situation of passive immunity involves adults with a deficiency in certain immune cells. In Immunoglobulin deficiency, they may have protection against some germs, but certain infections still threaten their health. If this is identified, a common treatment is infusion of immunoglobulin types that they lack, which then take up the fight on their behalf.

In our spiritual lives, especially as newborn Christians, we may not yet have developed resistance to some temptations. As we spend time in the Word of God and under the teaching of pastors and mature Christians, we learn to avoid or resist some things that we had no defense against on our own. This teaching and discipleship provide a framework by which we can defend against things we had not faced before.

All of us, when we are born again, move from death to life. As our souls are awakened, the Holy Spirit is with us, guiding us and defending us from enemy attacks of which we may not be fully aware. This 'passive immunity' is given to us, not requiring anything of us other than daily surrender in our walk with Christ. As Paul said in 1 Corinthians 2:12, "Now we have received, not the spirit of the world, but the Spirit who is from God, that we might know the things that have been freely given to us by God." Later in the same chapter, in verse 16, he goes on to say, "For 'who has known the mind of the Lord that he may instruct him?' But we have the mind of Christ." Talk about passive immunity! Through no effort of our own, we have access to the thoughts of Christ himself!

Auto-immune disease

Sometimes, our immune system goes awry, as in our patient, Anna, described at the beginning of this chapter. In this case, she has an autoimmune disorder in which her immune system attacks her own healthy tissue. This can be difficult to treat. In many cases, autoimmune disease is widespread as our immune cells circulate to all our organs. Treatment involves reducing the effectiveness of our immune response, which can make us susceptible to infection.

Spiritually, we sometimes interpret things in the wrong way and develop strong opinions protesting things that are not essential to our faith. In a sense, we attack our own body. This could be from subjecting ourselves to faulty teaching. If we suppress our 'immune system' by avoiding all teaching, that makes us susceptible to many other errors.

Immune deficiency

Rarely, a patient may be born with an immune deficiency. There were stories years ago of the boy in the plastic bubble, who had to wear a modified space suit when leaving the safety of the sterile home environment constructed for him. In this disease, Severe Combined ImmunoDeficiency, or SCID, patients are unable to mount a defense against even mild infections. Things that to most of us would be a mild annoyance can be fatal to those unable to fight back. Thankfully, a bone marrow transplant can provide the ability to manufacture those life-saving cells that defend us against pathogens.

Sometimes, an immune deficiency is acquired later in life. Probably the most well-known cause is HIV, or Human Immunodeficiency Virus. This virus attacks our infection-fighting cells, reducing certain protective cell lines to the point we develop AIDS, or Acquired ImmunoDeficiency Syndrome. Although perhaps not as severe as SCID, this still leaves its victims susceptible to infections that an intact immune system can easily fight off.

In the Body of Christ, I do not believe there is anything analogous to SCID. When we are born again, we receive the Holy Spirit, and as long as we follow Christ, and spend time in the Word and under the leadership of Pastors who preach the truth of the Bible, putting on the armor of God, we have supernatural protection at our disposal.

However, in an age of political correctness and tolerance, society seems to have turned to the belief that all religions lead to God, and that what we proclaim as 'our truth' should be honored and supported. The desire to avoid offending people who don't share our beliefs may leave us weakened in our own resolve to follow Christ. As we buy in to the societal trends, it may reduce our ability to fight off spiritual infections. Whether that be accepting unorthodox belief systems like those of the Latter Day Saints, or going overboard to support those in unbiblical relationships, or believing we are too wise to accept miraculous stories of the Bible as true, we are weakened spiritually.

It was Jesus, our Lord, who said, "I am the way, the truth, and the life. No one comes to the Father except through Me." (John 14:6) This is not a prideful opinion dreamed up by a church leader so we can claim to be superior to other belief systems. These are the 'red letters' of the Bible, spoken by Jesus. He proved His claims by submitting to the punishment that was meant for each of us and dying in our place. But He overcame death by rising on the third day. We must remember this above all else. This is what defines us as the Body of Christ. Everything else is secondary.

What's in a name?

Our patient, Anna Flaxus, refers to the deadly allergic reaction of anaphylaxis. Those with a specific allergy, for example peanuts or bee stings, may have such a strong reaction that it can be life-threatening. Even a tiny amount of the offending substance can cause the immune system to kick into overdrive, much like burning down the house to kill a spider. This 'nuclear attack' on the triggering offender causes widespread damage and danger. This sudden release of chemicals can cause circulatory shock, dropping the blood pressure to dangerously low levels, affecting all organs. The airway can swell, reducing the ability to take in oxygen. All of this can happen in seconds. The primary treatment for this frightening reaction is a quick injection of epinephrine followed by care in the nearest emergency department.

J. The Clinic: Those We Serve

Patients in this day and age have immediate and comprehensive access to information on virtually any topic related to their health. Sorting through this overwhelming volume of advice and opinion on every condition can be a daunting challenge. In addition to internet searches, direct-to-consumer advertising by way of television commercials invades our homes daily. It is a common occurrence in my practice for patients to bring in printouts of articles they found online, or to request specific labs or medications based on what they researched.

Most of these interactions are easily addressed when I provide information and explanation to them, explaining why such testing or treatment is not in their best interest. Unfortunately, strong opinions are becoming more common. Many patients come in fully convinced of information that medically is not wise or correct. They get this information from sources such as their uncle or best friend. Or they go to nontraditional sources that have training different than mainstream medicine, whether it be a naturopath, chiropractor, doula, acupuncturist, or others. Not to malign those professions, because they can be helpful and provide a valuable service to people, but sometimes the approach from such resources conflicts with the standard medical care that has developed through centuries of research and practice.

Some atypical recommendations are harmless, and we do not need to argue whether someone needs to take fourteen different vitamins and supplements. Medically, they offer little value, but arguing with a patient about them serves no purpose other than to alienate them and decrease the opportunity we may have to improve their health in other ways.

Other issues are more dangerous and fly in the face of proven medical care. The anti-vaccine movement needlessly places children at risk due to the unfounded belief that they cause harm, such as autism. This has been debunked, and the fraudulent research that launched this view has been retracted (**see chapter end note), but it remains on the internet forever. Similarly, those who opposed Covid vaccination decreased the chance of controlling such a deadly disease, yet I had many patients who bristled in anger when I suggested they get the Covid vaccine. Some even said they 'don't believe in Covid.'

Sometimes resistance to treatment is the result of a lack of understanding, and simply educating them or directing them to more trustworthy websites can help. Others avoid lifesaving procedures or recommended screening tests due to anxiety or fear. Counseling them on the risks and benefits of such tests can help, but fear is difficult to overcome.

Harmful behaviors and addictions have a way of relapsing repeatedly, and patients can fall into a cycle of resolving to quit drinking or to eating a healthy diet and exercising, only to place themselves in situations that sabotage their resolve. I also have a few patients who repeatedly allow their medication to lapse and do not follow up consistently. They even stop taking their insulin or blood thinners, which can be life-threatening. I must confess, I find myself getting irritated and frustrated when this happens. My (usually) inner dialogue runs along the lines of 'Why do you keep coming to me as your doctor if you will not do what I said you should do?' Then, I feel the conviction of the Spirit asking me the same question, as we read in Luke 6:46 (Why do you call me, 'Lord, Lord', and do not do what I say?)

Occasionally, legitimate risks that are very rare become exaggerated in the patient's mind and cause them to avoid proven treatments that are valuable. This may be a belief that statin medicine used for cholesterol reduction will cause liver failure, or that a proton pump inhibitor may cause dementia, or that a beta blocker medication for heart protection may cause impotence. Each of these concerns arises from a nugget of truth, but in each situation, the risk of this possible side effect or concern is extremely low, and the benefit of the therapy greatly outweighs any feared risk.

Those individuals who comprise the Body of Christ can have similar shortcomings and risky behaviors. Sometimes we seek spiritual information that contradicts orthodox doctrine or hold on to some new idea or practice from a 'fringe' source that detracts from our spiritual health. Many times we take our demands to God, expecting Him to bless what we have planned, rather than submitting to his will. Sometimes our fear prevents us from making spiritual progress. We exaggerate the possible difficulties we may face if God changes us.

In the case of patients disagreeing with my recommendations, I generally attempt to educate them and try to avoid needless arguments. My role is to recommend changes that can help them, but the responsibility lies with the patient. If someone decides against what I recommend, I do not want to sever the relationship. I hope they will continue to follow up so we can follow their health and continue to offer help, in the hope that they will eventually agree. Unfortunately, there are times the patients become angry and fracture the relationship on their end, or worse, begin to impact the care of other patients. Then we must ask them to find another doctor.

In the church, if people continue to attend services where they hear the truth of the Bible, the Holy Spirit has ongoing opportunities to open their eyes and convict them of the truth of what they hear. Rarely, though, they must be asked to leave if they refuse to hear and begin to negatively influence others.

** "Lancet retracts 12-year-old article linking autism to MMRIvaccines", from Canadian Medical Association Journal, 3/9/2010, found in National Library of Medicine, https://www.ncbi.nlm.nih.gov/pmc/articles/PMC2831678/

Other sources include The British Medical Journal, Nature Journal, Children's Hospital of Philadelphia, Mayo Clinic Health Systems, the New York Times, CNN, and others (as noted on a simple Google search of 'retraction of vaccine autism link')

11

Infection—Invaders

2 Peter 2:1 "But there were also false prophets among the people, even as there will be false teachers among you, who will secretly bring in destructive heresies, even denying the Lord who bought them, and bring on themselves swift destruction."

Titus Medea is 3 years old. His mother brings him to the office because he has had a fever and decreased appetite for the past two days. His nose has been running, and Mom saw him pulling on his left ear. When asked, she can only tell me she knows he had a fever because he felt warm, but his vital signs in the office confirm his temperature is 100.2 degrees Fahrenheit. On exam, his lungs are clear, and his throat is normal. However, his lymph nodes are swollen, and the left tympanic membrane (eardrum) is red and bulging, indicating infection. I prescribe an antibiotic and advise them to continue to treat the fever with Tylenol.

*****

Having a patient like this on my daily schedule can be nice because the history and exam are straightforward. The diagnosis can be quickly evident, and the treatment follows a well-worn path. It is not that I want people to suffer from infection, but unlike some of the other problems we see, this can be treated effectively the majority of the time.

Invasion

Infections are caused by foreign invaders that get into the tissues of the body and begin to grow, leading to an inflammatory response as our immune system gears up to fight off the foreign invader. This response can lead to fever and sometimes pain, as well as enlargement of lymph nodes in the area.

As a broad simplification, germs fall into two main categories-virus or bacteria. Of course, medicine is rarely that simple, and we sometimes must deal with infections due to a fungus or yeast organism, or other rare causes such as viral particles called prions (the cause of mad-cow disease).

Viral infections tend to be more diffuse, with body aches and fatigue being common symptoms. They may involve more than one body system, such as both vomiting and cough. The virus does not have the ability to reproduce itself, but it works by invading cells and using the body's own mechanisms to manufacture copies of its own genetic material. These copies then burst forth, moving to other cells or spreading to other hosts to continue their destructive work.

Bacterial infections tend to be more localized to a particular site or organ. This can affect just about any tissue in the body, from skin to kidney to lung to sinus to colon, and on and on. Usually, bacterial infections are more likely to have inflammatory changes like pus, redness, or warmth, and fever is more likely than with viral infections. Of course, there is some overlap of these generalizations.

Bacteria are complete cells with a nucleus and a cell wall, as well as various organelles needed for function. This gives them the ability to independently reproduce as they 'divide and conquer.' They do not typically invade and take over the cells of the body, but as they grow and spread, they may overwhelm the surrounding cells. As they consume resources for nutrition and growth, they may cause a localized infection like an abscess that can take up space and put pressure on the surrounding healthy tissue, impairing its function.

Spiritually, the Body of Christ may be infiltrated and invaded by outside influences. This may take the form of false teachings or unbiblical practices. It may be limited to a small group of members, or it may spread through the entire congregation. As Paul warned in 1 Corinthians 5:6: "Do you not know that a little leaven leavens the whole lump?" If it is not properly addressed and contained, this may threaten the life of the church, leaving it weakened and ineffective.

Some of these troubles are inflammatory and obvious, like bacterial infections that lead to fever, swelling, and redness. These invaders are not actually part of the body but instead enter with their own agenda. This could be false teachers or con men taking advantage of uninformed and immature believers. They may spread through the body, displacing the healthy members of the church and consuming resources so that the normal growth of the Body falters.

Others may be more subtle and diffuse, like a virus. They affect individual members, leading them to turn away from their normal healthy habits to spread their unhealthy practices. This may not initially be obvious, and it may even take the form of something morally neutral or even acceptable, but as it consumes more of the resources of church members, be it time, talent, or treasure, it can leave the body lethargic, achy, and feeling beat down. Spiritual appetite and activity may decrease. This fatigue and weakness keep us from actively reaching out or ministering to others.

Some infections do not remain localized, but instead find their way into the lymph channels or blood vessels and spread through the body. When infection becomes widespread, it is known as sepsis. This can be life-threatening, lowering blood pressure, overwhelming the organ function of the liver and the kidney, and surpassing the body's ability to maintain the status quo. Usually, this situation can be corrected with supportive care, strong intravenous doses of antibiotics, and treatment to maintain blood pressure and respiration.

When Moses was on Mount Sinai receiving the tablets of the Law from God Himself, the remainder of the camp was forming a golden calf and engaging in idol worship. This was not an isolated few, but the majority. This diffuse, widespread corruption is a form of spiritual sepsis. Removing the diseased and damaged tissue from the remaining healthy tissue can halt its spread, although the body is weakened and will take time to recover.

Another era of church history was the Reformation. The worldwide church had become corrupted ("septic") with indulgences, greed, and such. Martin Luther nailed his 95 theses to the door, beginning the recovery from this widespread spiritual infection.

Treatment

Treatment depends on the type of infection. Viral infections usually must run their course, and there are few anti-viral treatments. A few viral syndromes have medications that can help, such as herpes or chicken pox. Certain medications may help with influenza as well. But by and large, these do not kill the organisms that cause infection, unlike antibiotics that kill bacterial germs.

The primary treatment for bacterial infection is an antibiotic. The first antibiotic, penicillin, was discovered in 1928 when Alexander Fleming observed that the growth of his bacterial cultures was halted by contamination with a specific mold called

Penicillium. This discovery eventually led to the isolation of the antibiotic that was able to dramatically clear infections that previously had been fatal. Through the years, since penicillin was first discovered, many other antibiotics have been developed. They work on many different aspects of the bacterial structure and function.

Unfortunately, in this war, the germs fight back. Frequent exposure to an antibiotic allows bacteria to adapt and develop mechanisms of resistance that render them useless. Many news stories these days refer to the development of 'superbugs' or multi-drug-resistant bacteria that respond to few effective antibiotics. As newer drugs are developed to overcome resistance, many of them are exorbitantly priced, making them impractical for some patients. Thankfully, these infections are rare, and the commonly used antibiotics are generally effective.

Some bacterial infections fester and lead to a collection of pus known as an abscess. These can grow to be quite large and painful. Although antibiotics may kill the germs at fault, when there is such a large collection of infected material, they do not penetrate well. In such situations, surgical drainage of the abscess will allow quicker recovery.

In the Body of Christ, we sometimes face invaders that get a foothold, planting division that spreads deeply. This may overwhelm the ability of the local congregation to combat and heal. Something outside the body may be needed to conquer these invaders once they are established. Maybe an overseer or leader of the larger Church Body is needed, coming in to address false teachings, or even a surgical removal of a spiritual abscess.

Physically, treatment of bodily infections follows a stepwise pattern. First the immune system musters its troops to attack the invaders. If that fails, antibiotics are called upon to clear the infection. If the infection is entrenched and forms an abscess, surgical drainage or removal of the infected tissue may be required.

Similarly in the church, if someone offends us directly, the Bible gives guidelines on the sequential steps to take in order to address this before it becomes a more severe 'infection.' Matthew 18: 15-17 refers to these steps. "Moreover if your brother sins against you, go and tell him his fault between you and him alone. If he hears you, you have gained your brother. But if he will not hear, take with you one or two more, that 'by the mouth of two or three witnesses every word may be established.' And if he refuses to hear them, tell it to the church. But if he refuses even to hear the church, let him be to you like a heathen and a tax collector."

It may be that a false teacher has spent enough time in church settings that they know how to avoid detection or resist corrective actions. In this, they are much like the resistant bacteria described above. They may take such a strong hold on some members that they turn away from the offer of healing and restoration freely offered by God.

As Christians, we have our sure treatment in Christ. As David pleaded with God in Psalm 51, we can turn to Him with our sin, our 'infection,' and ask: 'Wash me thoroughly from my iniquity, and cleanse me from my sin'. (v 2) and 'Purge me with hyssop, and I shall be clean; wash me, and I shall be whiter than snow'. (v. 7)

Sexually Transmitted Infection

Unfortunately, human beings have a tendency to take risks, and our behavior may lead to infections. This is especially evident in my patients who come in for a 'regular STI check.'

Sexually transmitted infections (previously known as venereal disease—VD, then sexually transmitted diseases—STDs, and now as STIs) continue to wreak havoc on susceptible people. As our society has come to embrace sexual freedom in the past 60 years, the moral boundaries that helped curb promiscuous behavior have weakened. The traditional Christian values of abstinence until marriage and lifelong monogamy are viewed as archaic and restrictive by most in our society. We are fed a steady diet of entertainment that portrays 'normal' sexual behavior as sex early in a relationship, living together, casual relationships, same sex relationships, and risky sexual behaviors. As a result, we continue to have cases of sexually transmitted infections that are monitored at each state health department. HIV is not as newsworthy now, but it has not disappeared. Herpes is a chronic problem that many people treat as they get continued outbreaks. Syphilis has not been eradicated and continues to be a risk in certain populations. New treatments for viral hepatitis do not stop it from being spread, but help to control it after it is acquired. Gonorrhea, chlamydia, human papillomavirus, and others are still risks for those who do not practice what is commonly called 'safe sex.'

Despite these known and ongoing risks, I continue to have patients several times per year requesting routine STI screening. They are asymptomatic but recognize that their sexual behaviors have some risk, and they consider it being responsible to have a test now and then. I admit, this frustrates me, and it takes effort for me to keep from scolding them (sadly, I fail at this many times). I point out to them that there is no such thing as 'safe sex' outside the bonds of a solid, monogamous marriage. Condoms are not totally effective. If all we do is continue to check for infection while the risky behavior continues, eventually we will say, "Yep, there it is. You have [insert your favorite STI here]."

Just as in the discussion of STIs above, spiritually we are 'prone to wander' as the hymn describes. (Come Thou Fount of Every Blessing, written in 1758 by Robert Robinson, third verse). We follow the example of the children of Israel in returning to our sinful ways. And yet, if we return to the Great Physician, Jesus, he does not scold or turn us away. With mercy and grace, he forgives us, treats us, and points us in the right direction. Many times, we follow for a while and veer off course again.

The catholic church has a practice of confession. Although I am not catholic and have not studied this practice, it seems to me that many will depend on this each week, while it does not impact their daily behavior. A common saying is it is easier to ask forgiveness than permission, and the popular belief is that going to confession can excuse the sinful behavior in which they indulge. This ongoing exposure to spiritual 'infections' can and will eventually catch up with us, causing us to suffer things we could have avoided.

Prevention

Preventing infection is a much better option than battling to overcome an already-established infection. The tried-and-true method of handwashing and limiting direct contact with those who are ill can keep the germs from spreading to others. In the hospital setting, we sometimes need to wear masks, gowns, and gloves to limit the possible spread to other patients. With more dangerous infections that are difficult to treat, quarantine is still sometimes needed.

We can acquire infections in a variety of ways. Passively, we may just pass someone in the grocery store who sneezes, and we inhale the viral particles. Or if we have a scrape on our skin and come in contact with infected material, it can gain entry to our body and begin its work.

Many times, it is our own failures that leave us vulnerable. We may be in an environment that is rife with germs, and yet we fail to take precautions. Washing hands, wearing gloves, or face masks, or other personal protective equipment are vital in my work. If I become lax in these practices, infection risk grows, not just for me but for others that I encounter.

One of the most important tools in combating infection is immunization, as discussed in Chapter 10. Despite the unfortunate spread of misinformation about vaccines, they are proven to be safe and effective. Untold millions of lives have been spared by vaccination since the development of the smallpox vaccine by Edward Jenner in 1796. Now, we routinely vaccinate against a variety of viral and bacterial infections, including Measles, Mumps, Rubella, Chickenpox, Hepatitis B, Tetanus, Streptococcus Pneumoniae, Influenza, and many more.

As believers, we must be cautious with our exposures. Avoidance of sin is the safest option, as noted in 1 Thessalonians 5:22-"Abstain from every form of evil." Each of us may have a specific temptation to which we are susceptible. If it is alcohol or drugs, it would be unwise to intentionally spend time in environments where this is likely to occur. Likewise, if we have a weakness with gambling, going to dinner in a casino would be risky.

Psalm 1 describes a progression of walking in the counsel of the ungodly, then standing in the path of sinners, and finally sitting in the seat of the scornful. Each step of spending more time in ungodly, sinful, and scornful pursuits leads us further out of the path of righteousness.

The story of David and Bathsheba illustrates this. In 2 Samuel 11:1, we read "It happened in the spring of the year, at the time when kings go out to battle....But David remained at Jerusalem." He did not follow the appropriate behavior, and it led to exposure to temptation that pulled him into sin. Staying in Jerusalem was not sinful by itself, but that small step was on the path that ended with his sin.

For believers, our personal protective equipment is the armor of God. Ephesians 6 directs us to put on the whole armor of God. Verses 14-17 tell us this consists of the belt of truth, the breastplate of righteousness, covering our feet with the preparation of the gospel of peace, the shield of faith, and the helmet of salvation. In addition to covering ourselves with armor, we can go forth armed with the sword of the Spirit, which is the word of God.

Summary

As with physical infections, prevention of these spiritual infections is the safest course. Similar to wearing masks, gowns, and gloves, we must wear the spiritual armor listed in Ephesians 6 to protect ourselves. When an infection is recognized, we must limit our contact with it until we are protected by these garments. Preventing invasion by these outside influences is vital. Just as vaccines work by allowing our physical bodies to recognize foreign invaders before they can gain a foothold and begin to grow, we need steady exposure to the truth of God's word. This way, we can be so familiar with the truth that false teachings are obvious and can be avoided.

Although we in the body may sometimes be resistant to the cures available, thankfully, God can heal all diseases, restoring health to His Body on earth.

What's in a name?

The name of our young patient, Titus Medea, refers to his infection. Many kids will develop middle ear infections, which are known medically as 'Otitis Media.' The symptoms of pain in one (or both) ears and fever, as well as seeing a red, bulging eardrum, confirm the diagnosis. Thankfully, from my side of the otoscope, these are usually responsive to readily available treatments.

K. The Clinic: Sustenance

Each of us must ingest food and water each day to sustain our lives and health. We may survive several days without food and a few days without water in extreme circumstances, but our health will likely suffer. Daily nourishment and hydration are keys to good health and the prevention of disease.

In those unfortunate times of severe illness or life-threatening injury, among the first items of importance are hydration and nutrition. Without these, healing is nearly impossible. Most of the time, the priority of the paramedics or in the emergency room is to start an intravenous line (IV) with saline as quickly as possible. If someone is NPO (an abbreviation of the Latin term nil per os, meaning nothing by mouth) for more than three or four days, then they may receive TPN (total parenteral nutrition, meaning all calories by IV). The body needs nourishment and hydration to heal and to function properly.

Spiritually, the same is true. Visit almost any church long enough, and they will celebrate communion (sometimes known as the Lord's supper, or eucharist). The reason for this sacrament is to remind us of the Lord's sacrifice for us on the cross. Some congregations make this a part of worship every week, while others may participate monthly or quarterly. Whatever the frequency, communion is a routine part of worship. This was instituted by Jesus at the Last Supper. Luke 22:19-20 says, "And He took bread, gave thanks and broke it, and gave it to them, saying, 'this is My body which is given for you; do this in remembrance of Me.' Likewise, He also took the cup after supper, saying, 'This cup is the new covenant in My blood, which is shed for you.'"

Physically, there is no value to a tiny piece of cracker and a small serving of grape juice (assuming the reader does not believe in transubstantiation, where the elements are miraculously transformed into the body and blood of Jesus). However, as we regularly participate in this ritual, we are reminded again and again of God's love for us while we were yet sinners, sacrificing Himself to pay for our sins. We focus on his supply for our needs, and this reminder can strengthen our daily walk.

In a 'spiritual emergency,' where the Body is in danger of failing, the urgent need is to turn to God's supply, humbly turning back as we acknowledge our inability to save ourselves. It is the bodily sacrifice of Jesus (represented by the bread), and His blood shed for our forgiveness (symbolized by the juice), that are the only hope we have as believers. Without these, our spiritual life will steadily weaken and become unsustainable. In times where members of the Body have strayed and left the fellowship, if they return, this is, in a sense, a way of 're-membering,' or making them members again, of the Body of Christ.

In our daily walk, to preserve our spiritual health and guard against spiritual decline, we must steadily partake of spiritual nutrition and hydration. I picture this as a daily 'diet' of the Word of God, and daily 'drinking in' the Spirit through prayer. In these activities, we connect with God, and our spiritual body, individually and collectively, remains strong.

Just as we need daily calories to maintain physical function, it is the daily communion with God that keeps us from becoming weak and ineffective spiritually. We cannot store up our spirituality on Sunday and ignore it the rest of the week if we hope to remain healthy. God continues to supply our daily needs now, just as he supplied the daily manna during the Exodus.

12

Cancer—Pride

Proverbs 14:30 "A sound heart is life to the body, but envy is rottenness to the bones."

Karsyn Ozhenyk is 52 years old. He presents to the office with a lump in his neck. He noticed this several months ago, and his wife just found out about it. She scheduled the appointment for him. This lump is in the front of his neck, just above his collarbone on the right side. It is not tender. He thinks it may be slowly growing over time.

Examination shows no other findings other than a firm nodule in the area of the right thyroid lobe. There is a small nodule palpable just lateral to this as well. He does not smoke currently, but smoked a pack per day until he quit five years ago. The history is otherwise unremarkable until he mentions growing up in southern Ukraine. He remembers the news about the Chernobyl disaster when he was a teenager and knows some of his relatives developed health problems over the following decades.

Laboratory levels are normal, but a sonogram shows a suspicious tumor on the thyroid gland, and a needle biopsy confirms cancer cells. I refer him to a surgeon as well as an oncologist to discuss further treatment.

*****

Cancer comes in many forms. It can occur in any type of tissue in the body and cause any number of symptoms (or none at all), depending on location and size. Despite the variations, however, all cancers are the same in one respect. A single cell or type of tissue enters an abnormal growth phase that does not respond to typical limits placed on it by the body's control systems. The cells have mutated such that they have an abnormal appearance under the microscope. As this unfettered growth continues, it disrupts the tissue around it, displacing it and preventing it from normal function. It consumes calories, causing weight loss and weakness. It must be removed or destroyed in order to stop this rampant growth and destruction.

Some cancers can be obvious. For example, certain skin cancers are visible and destructive. The 'rodent ulcer' of basal cell cancer can cause a large, ulcerated lesion on the skin where it occurs. Thankfully, it does not often spread, but the localized destruction can be dramatic. Excising this affected skin, being sure to allow for adequate margins around it, can be curative.

Other cancers are much more subtle and can mimic other, more common ailments. Stomach pain may be more likely to be gastritis or ulcers, but if it does not respond to usual treatment, imaging may reveal a tumor in the pancreas that is already too advanced to remove or even treat effectively.

Surgeons are well-trained in removing abnormal tissues, being sure to allow enough normal margin around the tumors to hopefully be curative. However, it only takes one cancer cell that spreads to a lymph node for it to begin conquering new tissues. Oncologists are constantly developing fresh treatment protocols to kill rapidly growing cancer cells without destroying the normal healthy cells of the body. Radiation oncologists are expert snipers, targeting cancerous tissue without disturbing adjacent cells. It is an ongoing battle.

Me First

At the heart of spiritual cancer is self-centeredness. In our modern society, the whole concept of 'looking out for number one' seems to be the top priority. We easily forget the One Who should be number one in our lives. Once we turn our focus inward on ourselves, we begin to lose our sensitivity to the needs of others. We grab the things we want before others can take them. We cry 'Unfair!' when our perceived rights are slighted. We do not fully believe the promise of Philippians 4:19: "And my God shall supply all your need according to His riches in glory by Christ Jesus."

Envy—Why do YOU get to do that and not me?

The evil twins of spiritual cancer are envy and pride. Envy focuses on the success of others and desires it for ourselves instead. It is not so much hoping to do as well as someone else, but rather to do better than them. I remember a speaker once referring to the fact that the popular magazine is not 'Homes and Gardens" but rather "BETTER Homes and Gardens." We want our stuff to be better than that of our neighbors, and if we can't have it, neither should they.

In the church, this can begin to take hold in leadership roles. Watching a soloist sing in a Sunday service, we may stop focusing on the message of the music and instead think, "I can do better than that!" Or ballots to elect church board members may exclude us.

Seeking a role God has not designed for us will not lead to profitable ministry.

Paul addresses this in 1Corinthians 12:12-31. His humorous take on body parts envying each other leads to absurdity. "If the whole body were an eye, where would be the hearing? And if the whole were hearing, where would be the smelling?.... If they were all one member, where would the body be?" (The answer, my friends, is 'dead'!) Verse 25-26, sums it up, saying 'that there should be no schism in the body, but that the members should have the same care for one another. And if one member suffers, all the members suffer with it; or if one member is honored, all the members rejoice with it." I am afraid that in many church bodies, however, we still have the unfortunate situation where the nose runs, and the feet smell, instead of the other way around. Neither outcome is desirable.

Pride—Look what I get to do! Don't you wish you were me?

Similarly, pride also takes the focus off God's work in us and promotes our own work and accomplishments. When one spiritual 'cell' seeks his or her own rights and privileges above those around them, it may only be a localized problem. However, unchecked, they may inflate their own importance or role and not respond to the corrections set forth in Scripture. If this person is in a leadership role, they can draw others under their own influence and may consume resources needed for ministry. I envision TV preachers soliciting donations, which they use to fund their own mansions or jets. This may not simply look bad, but can also destroy the faith of those looking on who assume that it is an accurate reflection of Christianity in general.

I believe that the root of all sin is pride. Pride promotes what I want over what others say. It is putting myself first. It is saying I know better than God, that if I eat of the fruit of the tree, I will not surely die (Genesis 3:4). It is believing that I created my own success and 'deserve' everything I desire to have. It is setting myself up as my own king, refusing to bow the knee to the King of all Kings.

Unless we acknowledge our own inadequacy, confessing our sins, feeling the weight of guilt that turns us toward God, we cannot become children of God. But that is just the beginning. In a very real sense, we must 'take up our cross daily,' dying to our own desires. We must strive to be outward-focused followers of Christ (the mission statement of my own local church). I am well aware in my own life how easy it is for my focus to shift away from God and to myself. We need to daily remind ourselves that His is the kingdom and the power and the glory forever. It is not ours.

This 'spiritual cancer' can afflict any individual who does not submit to the limits and controls which God provides.

Treatment

There are many treatments for cancer, depending on the type and location. New treatments are becoming available every year, with great optimism for each. Whether it be chemotherapy, radiation, surgery, or targeted immune therapy, each option offers specific benefits to specific types of cancer. The more systemic the therapy, like chemotherapy that circulates all through the bloodstream searching for rapidly growing cells, the more likelihood of widespread side effects. Researchers constantly seek a 'magic bullet' that will target cancer cells while leaving healthy cells alone, thus reducing toxicity.

In the Body of Christ, targeting the cancer of envy and pride is very focused. The Holy Spirit speaks directly to us, convicting us of our prideful self-centeredness. There may be hundreds of people hearing a sermon, but the word of God is living and active, even when spoken, and the same words may leave many unaffected, while those of us diseased by specific sins may feel that familiar heart pounding and regret that leads us to repentance. At each worship service, there may be cells of the Body being treated while their seatmates have no idea. This may not be a 'magic bullet,' but it is supernaturally targeted therapy.

Summary

Spiritual cancer can begin subtly when we compare our situations to those of others, but if we allow this to grow unchecked, it may lead to envy or pride. This is especially displayed on social media as we share the perfect version of life as we wish it to be. Even if we add "#blessed" to each post, it seems clear that the motivation of many is pride, hoping to incite envy in others.

We must recognize that all we have is from God. 'For by grace you have been saved through faith, and that not of yourselves; it is the gift of God, not of works, lest anyone should boast." (Ephesians 2:8-9) And we must remember that "God shall supply all your needs according to His riches in glory by Christ Jesus." (Philippians 4:19) We don't need to covet what others have since God will provide for us in a way that is specific to our need. These reminders help us resist the cancers of envy and pride in the Body of Christ.

What's in a name?

Karsyn Ozhenyk refers to substances that are carcinogenic. This term means they are capable of causing cancer. Obvious carcinogens may be cigarettes or radiation exposure, as in the case of Karsyn described above. There are many chemicals we may encounter throughout our lives, whether they be in cleaning products or processed foods, or workplace exposures. Most of us are subjected daily to the sun's ultraviolet rays, which can promote skin cancers. Radon can be in basements all over the Midwest. Despite this widespread exposure, God has created natural protective protocols in our tissues and cells that can limit these harmful effects. As a physician, I must remind you to schedule routine physical check-ups so recommended screening tests can be ordered.

L. The Clinic: Where Is Our Focus?

Many times, a patient comes in worried that they are not losing weight. They have been exercising and watching their diet consistently, and they notice their clothes fitting more loosely, and that they have better endurance and strength, but the weight is not budging. In this situation, I try to redirect their focus to the fact that they are getting healthier. They have better exercise tolerance and strength, and they are slimming down. The number on the scale is only one measure of their health. Many remain frustrated or even depressed by this.

Others will come in for follow-up a few months later than we recommended, having run out of their supply of medications weeks ago. Most of them are quick to apologize to me for not following up. Again, I must shift their focus. It is not my health, but theirs that is suffering. There is no need to apologize to me, but I hope they will understand the importance of continuing medications and doing regular follow-up as it pertains to their own health.

I remember years ago, a young man about to go off to college saw me for a physical. In the course of our discussion, he asked me how he could use drugs safely while he was in college. Talk about wrong focus! He told me very frankly that he knew he would use drugs and just wanted to make sure he did it in a safe way. I suppose in some ways it was good that he was at least aware that there were dangers, but in this case, his mind was pretty firmly made up. I hope he is still doing ok!

There are plenty of examples. Some take as many as fifteen supplements and vitamins daily, but when I recommend a prescription, they are adamant that they don't want to take medicine.

Others want medication or surgery to lose weight, so they don't have to work on it themselves. Even healthy habits like running can become an obsession, and many marathon runners begin to get knee and hip pain, or suffer dehydration and muscle injury, as they remain proud of their health.

Spiritually, we can also lose focus. We follow good practices like tithing or Bible reading, but it becomes more habitual than meaningful. We flip through the scriptures and choose a verse at random, skimming it as we mentally check off that duty for the day. Yes, these are good things for Christians to do, but even good things can be done without involving our hearts.

Through the centuries, the church has revered things related to Jesus or to the Saints of old. Some, especially the Catholic church, have accumulated relics, whether it be the famed shroud of Turin, or bones reported to be those of Zaccheus. One website even reports there were claims to have the 'holy foreskin' of the infant Jesus, although it has gone missing! (15 Weird and Wonderful Religious Relics | J.F.Penn (jfpenn.com))

In Acts 8:18-19, Simon the sorcerer attempted to buy the power to lay hands on people so they could receive the Holy Spirit. That sounds like a good thing to do, doesn't it? But Peter rebuked him (vv 20-23), saying he was "poisoned by bitterness and bound by iniquity." Doing spiritual, or even Holy things for self-centered reasons will not help the health of the Body of Christ.

In Mark 5:25-34, we read the story of the woman who had been ill for twelve years. (Verse 26 is probably my least favorite Bible verse, stating that she had "suffered many things from many physicians. She had spent all that she had and was no better, but rather grew worse." But I digress.) In her faith, she knew Jesus could heal her. She braved the large crowd, pushing her way through to touch the hem of his garment, trying to 'steal a blessing.' Jesus immediately identified what happened and did not allow her to remain in the shadows. I believe part of the reason for this was to clarify that what is important is Jesus, not the things around him.

Psalm 16:11 says, "You will show me the path of life; in Your presence is fullness of joy; at Your right hand are pleasures forevermore." I think sometimes we selfishly focus so much on the pleasures in God's right hand that the more important things are out of focus, such as His presence. In His most famous sermon, the one on the mount, Jesus instructs us to "seek first the kingdom of God and His righteousness, and all these things shall be added to you." It is important to focus on what is most important.

In our worship, we sing a lot of songs about the name of Jesus. The Word of God instructs us to pray in the name of Jesus, to baptize in the name of Jesus, and anoint the sick in the name of the Lord. Philippians 2:9-11 tells us:

"Therefore God also has highly exalted Him and given Him the name which is above every name, that at the name of Jesus every knee should bow, of those in heaven, and of those on earth, and of those under the earth, and that every tongue should confess that Jesus Christ is Lord, to the glory of God the Father."

Yes, the name of Jesus is wonderful, matchless, and above every name. However, in this day and age, I fear we lose the meaning of this. Doing things 'in the name' of Jesus implies we are doing them as His representative. It is not an incantation to tack on to our prayers to coerce God to provide what we want. The verses above are an indication of the power of Jesus Himself, such that even the mere mention of His name reveals His glory, shining a light on our own unworthiness.

When singing, I focus a lot on lyrics more than tunes (that is why certain songs bug me, like the line 'The same power that rose Jesus from the dead…' being grammatically incorrect; or—I share this with some embarrassment—The First Noel. Does anyone else feel like the lyrics are clunky and forced to match the tune? But once again I digress—you can see my lack of focus in this section on focus!!). Recently, in church, we were singing about the name of Jesus, and there was a line that bothered me. I found myself singing with the rest of the congregation, "You are worthy of Your Name." It struck me as odd that we, mere mortals, are telling Jesus that he lives up to the name.

When I hear someone say they are worthy to call themselves something, the implication is that the name is the ultimate goal, and we have decided they are good enough to claim it. In the case of Jesus, I think we get that backwards. He is the ultimate, the pinnacle. He has many names, including Wonderful, Counselor, Mighty God, Everlasting Father, Prince of Peace, Alpha, Omega, King of Kings, Lord of Lords, Lily of the Valley. Sorry if I offend someone, but I think it is more that the name Jesus is worthy of Him!

When we focus on things that are around Jesus, or part of Him, or on His name—anything other than Jesus Himself—in some ways it seems we are seeking something for ourselves. We want healing, or power, or importance. By reaching for the hem of His garment in the crowd, we are insulated and doing something for ourselves. But when we truly encounter Him, we are humbled and laid bare. The light of his glory shines on anything we try to keep in the shadows. And He loves us and heals us and provides pleasures forevermore if we will seek Him and His kingdom first.

13

Diabetes—Lifestyle

James 1:22 "But be doers of the word, and not hearers only, deceiving yourselves."

Alice Flangrans is 52 years old and comes in for regular follow-up. Since I saw her a year ago, she has been much less active and, as a result, has gained eighteen pounds. For the past month, she has experienced episodes of blurred vision and has noticed a burning sensation in her toes when she lays down at night. I order routine blood tests, and they reveal that her glucose is 422. I order an additional test called hemoglobin A1c, and it is 13.2, indicating uncontrolled diabetes (normal being 5.7 or less). I start her on metformin and refer her to the diabetes educators to begin a regimen of diet and exercise, instructing her to return in three months to recheck her labs.

*****

What is it? How do I get it?

Diabetes, in basic terms, is an inability to process glucose. This can be due to a lack of production of insulin in the pancreas, also known as Type 1 diabetes, but for this discussion, we are concerned with Type 2 diabetes. In this case, we become desensitized to the insulin we produce. This is largely hereditary, with family members passing it on to subsequent generations, but obesity is a common risk factor. As we accumulate body fat, our resistance to insulin increases, allowing glucose to circulate at higher-than-normal levels despite still producing insulin.

If this problem is identified early enough, there may be no symptoms or complications. This is one reason regular physical check-ups are important. In decades past, a diagnosis of 'sugar' (as some knew it) was accompanied by fear of inevitably losing eyesight, having a foot amputated, and ending up on dialysis. Thankfully, with regular exams and screening blood work, these are exceedingly rare complications of diabetes today. Earlier detection and lifestyle changes, as well as more effective and better-tolerated medications, bring much better control of diabetes and therefore prevent these dreaded consequences.

Spiritually, problems may be similarly passed from parents to their children. If our physical families are lax in spiritual matters, we sometimes follow those same practices, skipping church when there is a big game on, or settling for watching worship services online instead of participating in fellowship with others. Spending time with fellow believers, worshipping together, can help us stay spiritually healthy. The regular Sunday morning spiritual 'checkup' can help identify and correct early problems before they take hold (as discussed in chapter one).

Just as obesity has become epidemic in the United States in recent years, I get a sense there is also widespread spiritual obesity. We are fed a rich spiritual diet every Sunday, but we do not exercise spiritually. As we get comfortable in our own ways, we become resistant to good Biblical doctrine, much like a diabetic is resistant to insulin. As this continues, we become susceptible to spiritual complications that in many ways mirror the physical complications of diabetes.

The best way to help prevent early diabetes and avoid complications is to change our diet and exercise. As we eat healthy foods, limiting carbohydrates and sugars, we reduce the levels of glucose that must be controlled. As we exercise, we use up the circulating sugar before it gets deposited.

Spiritually, diet and exercise are also vital to health. A diet of the meat of the Word of God can give life to the spiritual body. Exercising the spiritual disciplines strengthens the Body of Christ. As each of us participates in spiritual exercises like prayer, Bible study, and evangelism, and as we run the race with perseverance, we stave off spiritual obesity that threatens our health.

What's the problem with a little sugar? Complications

You may wonder why a little extra sugar can be so dangerous. Grossly simplified, as glucose accumulates in our bloodstream, it impacts nerves and blood vessels. Since every part of our body has these structures, diabetes potentially can impact almost every aspect of our health.

Consider just a few of our organ systems:

Vision

Our eyes have many small, fragile capillaries providing blood supply to the retina, where our sight originates. As glucose remains uncontrolled, these may leak protein material or, even worse, have small hemorrhages. This disrupts the sensitive tissue of the retina, preventing us from sensing the images in front of us. As the damage of diabetic retinopathy progresses unchecked, blindness results.

Spiritually, as we spend time in church, not exercising, becoming spiritually obese, our awareness of the needs around us may dim. Eventually, spiritual blindness makes us unable to perceive, and we lose God's vision of reaching the lost and hurting we encounter each day.

Feet

Our extremities may begin to lose sensation as the delicate nerve cells furthest from our brains are rendered ineffective by excess sugar. As we lose sensation, this is sometimes replaced by a burning sensation in our feet that can be very painful. This is called neuropathy. As we have less sensation, simple everyday occurrences, like developing a blister or stepping on a Lego brick, can lead to injuries that we don't feel, and therefore, we continue to bear weight on this area instead of limping to offload continued pressure. As the sore increases in diameter and depth, bacteria can invade, leading to infection. The blood vessels to this area may not provide adequate circulation to bring lifesaving infection-fighting cells to join the battle. As the infection progresses to gangrene, it could invade the bone, leading to bone infection, known as osteomyelitis, which is difficult to clear. Unfortunately, there are still patients who require amputations of one toe after another until eventually the foot is lost. Thankfully, this is rare.

We in the Church commonly refer to ourselves as the hands and feet of Jesus (although we usually don't consider what actually happened to His hands and feet on the cross). If we grow lazy in our walk with Christ, we may grow numb. Even if our vision is still intact, we may see needs around us but become callused and unable to feel for the lost and hurting. This progressive insensitivity in the Body of Christ causes harm and may lead to spiritual infections, as discussed in Chapter 10. As Paul said in Ephesians 6:15, we must protect our feet with the preparation of the gospel of peace. This is part of our preparation to "withstand in the evil day, and having done all, to stand." (Ephesians 6:13). Without this preparation and protection, spiritual neuropathy may progress, leaving us unable to stand.

Kidneys

Our kidneys are vital to maintaining our health. They provide acid-base balance, blood pressure control, electrolyte balance, and regulate many nutrients and medications. There is an amazingly intricate network of capillaries that are vital to these functions. Unchecked diabetes, though, can damage these blood vessels. As this occurs, they become much less efficient at filtering impurities and maintaining balance. We are blessed to live in an era where dialysis can supply the function that has been lost as kidney failure progresses, but the large, technically advanced machines used in dialysis are not nearly as effective as our twin marvels of creation that silently function for most of us throughout our lives without our conscious awareness.

We discussed kidney function as it relates to the Body of Christ in a previous chapter. In cases of spiritual 'kidney failure,' our spiritual discernment (analogous to our kidneys) wanes, and we are not able to test everything in light of scripture, holding on to the good. This lack of discernment can leave us susceptible to poor doctrine and to poor spiritual nutrition. In turn, we become unable to fight spiritual infections. We may become more caustic in our dealings with others as our ability to control our spiritual blood pressure and acidity is lost.

Stomach

Our stomach carries out its function under the direction of our autonomic nervous system (described in an earlier chapter), controlling our sensation of fullness and the processing of nutrients through our digestive tract. When diabetes is uncontrolled for too long, it may disrupt this movement of food and emptying of our stomachs. People with gastroparesis, or slowed emptying of the stomach, suffer nausea and vomiting with loss of appetite. This can be miserable.

With spiritual diabetes, the Body of Christ may likewise lose spiritual appetite. We stay constantly full of spiritual junk food, taking away our hunger and thirst for righteousness. Our nutrition fades, and we become weakened and unable to function at our best.

Weight Loss

For patients with type II diabetes, weight loss is one of the mainstays of treatment. Even for those without diabetes, weight loss is a major concern for many people, sometimes to the point of depression. Very commonly, patients will see me asking for help to lose weight. Some will ask about the latest diet trend they have heard about. Most of them ask for medication to expedite this process. Some have gone to weight loss clinics or researched weight loss surgery as well.

My first response typically is that the only way to lose weight consistently is to increase exercise and decrease calorie intake. Of course, it can be more complex with issues of insulin resistance or medications that impact weight, but diet and exercise remain the mainstay of healthy habits that help to control weight. The effectiveness of this has been dramatically displayed on the television show The Biggest Loser which aired for several seasons beginning in 2004. Despite the unfortunate name, many of the contestants lost significant amounts of weight, many more than half of their initial body weight, through a regimen of intense exercise and strict diet supervised by their team leaders.

While it is true that people may lose weight following a specific diet plan, this is likely to be short-lived if they do not also change their lifestyle around eating behaviors. Similarly, there are medications that can be very effective as adjunct treatments, but an appetite suppressant is only effective as long as it is continued. They are not intended to be chronic, and once they are stopped, weight maintenance depends on following a healthy diet and exercising. Even among contestants on The Biggest Loser, follow-up studies showed that most regained their weight after the controlled environment of the show ended.

Short-term spiritual emphases like Bible Study groups or revival meetings can help us grow closer to the Lord, but this may not last long if we do not follow a healthy spiritual lifestyle of 'diet and exercise.' Daily time in Bible reading and prayer, as well as following healthy spiritual habits, such as being faithful in church attendance and tithing, assist us in ongoing spiritual growth.

Spiritually, many of us seek a quick answer to overcoming temptation and growing in our relationship with the Lord. We do not like the pain and hardship that are brought on by trials and hard things in our lives, and we try to avoid them, but if we have been in a church environment for more than a few years, we have very likely heard a pastor tell us that these are the times we see great spiritual growth.

Just as patients seek an appetite suppressant to reduce hunger so they can lose weight, many of us want a spiritual 'appetite suppressant' to take away our hunger for worldly things. We can't follow shortcuts and avoid our own responsibilities in either our physical or our spiritual health if we want to continue to grow and thrive in each realm. To be clear, our efforts will not save us. That is the work of God through the sacrifice of Jesus and the help of the Holy Spirit. But Paul wrote in 1 Corinthians 9: 24, "Do you not know that those who run in a race all run, but one receives the prize? Run in such a way that you may obtain it.", and in verse 27 of the same chapter, "But I discipline my body and bring it into subjection, lest, when I have preached to others, I myself should become disqualified."

Treatment

These are but a few of the widespread troubles we may face if diabetes goes unchecked. However, if identified early and if we follow a regimen of diet and exercise and weight loss along with proper medications, most patients are able to control diabetes and stave off these possible complications.

For the Body of Christ, the first step, as with many spiritual problems, is to improve our 'diet and exercise.' The spiritual disciplines give us structure in our spiritual lives and lead to healthy activities and focus on proper spiritual nutrition. As we exercise, even if we start with basic Bible reading, church attendance, and prayer, we will begin to see improvement in our condition.

Many of the medicines used to treat diabetes physically are designed to improve how our body's tissue naturally functions, thereby improving control of sugar levels and avoiding complications. Similarly, God uses things outside ourselves to improve our spiritual health. Proper teaching of scripture and spiritual leadership from pastors and mentors can be vital to our spiritual health.

Summary

Physically, diabetes has the potential to impact almost every organ of our body, causing widespread havoc if not identified and treated. It is closely aligned with obesity and lack of exercise.

As the Body of Christ, we may also suffer from spiritual obesity if we do not pursue good nutrition and participate in spiritual exercise. As we are faithful in our gathering together, we may identify problems early before they cause complications that weaken the Body of Christ.

What's in a name?

Our patient in this chapter is Alice Flangrans. If you say it fast enough, it sounds a little like "islets of Langerhans." This anatomical tissue consists of clusters ('islets') of endocrine cells in the body of the pancreas. In the chapter on the gastrointestinal system, we discussed the exocrine function of the pancreas in digestion, but these islet cells provide the endocrine (hormonal) function. They produce insulin and glucagon, which aid in balancing the glucose levels circulating through our body.

M. The Clinic: Payments

A major influence in medicine today is cost. In America, most people have health insurance. This has been a political emphasis in recent years, with a push for everyone to have coverage to some degree. For those without an insurance plan, it only takes one hospital admission to accumulate thousands of dollars in debt. A quick Google search indicates that as of 2021, the overall burden of medical debt in the United States was approximated at $220 billion.

Many of my patients, especially as they age, may need ten, fifteen, or twenty medications (or more) as their health declines. Without insurance coverage, this can be a very large expense, and some are forced to decide which of their prescribed medications are most important as they balance other household expenses.

With insurance coverage, the burden is much lower. Many patients come into the office for an appointment at the first sign of a sniffle. Some who are more anxious may come in every couple of weeks with new concerns that only require reassurance. They are not bothered by health care costs since they have a very low copay for each visit. Others, however, struggle to pay even a moderate copay when they really need to be seen. Fear of high costs can be a deterrent to necessary care.

In certain situations, the medical bill is paid by someone other than the patient. A victim of a car accident caused by someone else, or an employee making a workers' compensation claim, bears no cost. The entire bill is covered by the driver or company responsible for their injury. In such cases, threats of litigation may greatly escalate medical charges as more tests are ordered to satisfy legal counsel that nothing was left out of their care. The patient typically does not care since they have no responsibility to cover the cost. Unfortunately, the legal system seems to be a strong factor in driving up health care costs as doctors attempt to reduce their liability by ordering extra tests to avoid lawsuits.

From a spiritual standpoint, we all carry a deadly burden of sin debt. None of us can pay for this ourselves. We are born already having a sinful nature, and as we follow our own desires, we continue to travel the broad way that leads to destruction.

Throughout history, the goal of religion has been to satisfy this debt in God's eyes. Whether it be ancient religions sacrificing to pagan gods, Muslims striving to please Allah and doing a pilgrimage to Mecca, Jews striving to follow a myriad of laws, or Mormons striving to do good, all share the common problem of trying to do enough good to balance the bad in our lives.

The Bible is clear that this is impossible in our own strength. We read:

All have sinned and fall short of the glory of God (Romans 3:23)

There is none righteous, no, not one. (Romans 3:10)

Every one of them has turned aside; they have together become corrupt; there is none who does good. No, not one (Psalms 53:3)

But we are all like an unclean thing. And all our righteousnesses are like filthy rags; (Isaiah 64:6)

But we also have hope. God's word reminds us:

…the gift of God is eternal life in Christ Jesus our Lord. (Romans 6:23)

For by grace you have been saved through faith, and that not of yourselves; it is the gift of God (Ephesians 2:8)

Be still and know that I am God (Psalms 46:10)

And the words of Jesus to those who are striving to save themselves: Come to Me, all you who labor and are heavy laden, and I will give you rest. (Matthew 11:28)

The truth is, none of us is capable of paying our own spiritual debt. While we may count ourselves more righteous than others around us, we are still filthy. If our command was to jump across the Grand Canyon, some of us could jump higher or farther than others, but it is ludicrous to think any of us could jump that far. Just like in the operating room, the surgeon puts on clean clothes and washes his hands, but is still not sterile without the covering of the sterile surgical gowns and gloves. His efforts are not enough.

The good news of the Gospel is that our debt has been paid. We don't even have a copay. None of us contributes to our own salvation. We just accept the free gift of God's sacrifice on our behalf. This is the amazing grace of which we sing.

Since we bear no cost, we are free to bring all of our concerns to God, no matter how small. Hebrews 4:16 instructs us: "Let us therefore come boldly to the throne of grace, that we may obtain mercy and find grace to help in time of need." (NKJV)

At times, pride will stop someone from accepting 'charity,' worried it will make them feel inadequate or weak. Instead, they continue striving, working, laboring, wearing themselves out to pay a debt they cannot keep up with. Spiritually, our pride in our own strength of character, or our humanistic belief that we all can work together to save our human race, may stop some from believing that their efforts will never be enough. They refuse to admit their bankruptcy in God's eyes.

14

Organ Transplants—Change of Leadership

Ezekiel 36:26 "I will give you a new heart and put a new spirit within you; I will take the heart of stone out of your flesh and give you a heart of flesh."

Lynn Farmer is 47. She comes in with a lump on her neck that has been growing. It is not painful, but continues to enlarge. With further questioning, she has noticed fatigue, night sweats, and some unintentional weight loss. On exam, her vital signs are ok, but her BMI is only 20, and she has lost 21 kg since her last visit eight months ago. She has a large lump on the right side of her neck that is visible from across the room. It measures seven centimeters, and there is another smaller one adjacent to it. A chest X-ray is ordered and shows adenopathy (lymph node enlargement) around the central chest structures. I refer her to an Otolaryngologist (an ear, nose, and throat specialist), and his biopsy confirms high-grade lymphoma. She undergoes treatment by oncology, but with limited response. She is then sent to the local transplant center to be evaluated for a bone marrow transplant.

*****

As we have discussed, all our body's systems are susceptible to illness and injury that can compromise function. Thankfully, the majority of these troubles respond to treatment. Unfortunately, the risk of irreversible damage remains.

In 1 Corinthians 12:26, Paul comments that in the Church body, "..if one member suffers, all the members suffer with it…". This literally occurs when damage accumulates in our bodies. As one organ fails, this multiplies the stress on the rest of the body, creating a snowball effect of worsening function in each of our organs, making life unsustainable. When this happens, few medical options remain.

For more than a century, doctors have toyed with taking an organ from one person and transplanting it to another. In the early 1900s, doctors in Europe, caring for patients dying of renal failure, attempted transplants with kidneys from monkeys or goats. These attempts universally failed within a few days. (see www.history.com/news/organ-transplants-a-brief-history, accessed January 16, 2022).

The first successful kidney transplant was in 1956 between identical twins. It wasn't until four years later that researchers found ways to prevent rejection of donated organs with immunosuppressants. Then, the race was on.

Since 1966, in addition to the kidneys, transplant surgeries have been performed for pancreas, liver, heart, heart-lung, single lung, double lung, intestines, partial liver, hand, partial face, full face, legs, and penis. Aside from these organs, bone marrow is commonly transplanted, and cornea transplants have been restoring sight to people since 1905. I'm sure there are others, but this is quite an amazing list!

Early in this journey, most donated organs were harvested from patients who had recently died, but by 2001, the total number of living donors exceeded the number of deceased.

Of course, aside from the surgical techniques and treatment of rejection, great advancements have been made in preserving the donated organs before transplant, national coordination of donor registries to connect patients in need with suitable donors, and life-sustaining measures for those with organ failure to extend survival until organs are available.

For most recipients, life is dramatically improved. Of course, they must regularly follow up with the physicians and be alert for any sign of rejection, but most consider this a reasonable price to pay for extending their life span.

Living donors also must make some concessions. After someone sacrificially donates a kidney (like my wife), life can be completely normal, but without the backup system of a second kidney, any mild insult to the one remaining could be problematic. Being diligent to watch for urinary tract infections or stones, and avoiding non-steroidal anti-inflammatory medications are advised.

Similarly, we have seen many ways the Body of Christ can suffer injury or failure. The majority of these are healed by God as the person involved repents and restores damaged relationships. Unfortunately, this does not always happen.

Major moral failures seem to occur all too often. TV evangelists have made national headlines many times when their sins come to light. Sadly, instead of being praised for their ministry to the Kingdom of God, we associate names like Jimmy Swaggart, Jim Bakker, and Ted Haggard with moral failures that led to public disgrace. Likewise, sexual abuse by catholic priests seems to have become a common story in the media. Just Google 'moral failures of pastors', and you will find many sad examples.

When failure of leadership is severe, as discussed in the chapter on orthopedic problems, this can cripple the church. In certain situations, the best remedy is to remove the 'damaged organ' and transplant a healthy replacement.

The bible refers to a type of spiritual transplant in Ezekiel 36:26, the verse quoted at the beginning of this chapter.

Donor

As in physical organ transplants, the spiritual transplant, many times, is supplied by a 'living donor.' Someone in a leadership position at one church is called to assume the leadership position that was abandoned by failure in another. In the case of a healthy donor church, it will continue to thrive, and in many cases may support the one who was called away.

Of course, there remains a risk that some supporters of this transplanted leader may be hurt. Some may stop attending church and become weakened in their walk. Others may follow them to the new assignment, also potentially weakening the donor church. In such situations, maintaining focus on Christ and His Kingdom should supersede focus on human personality.

Cadaver donations are still common and remain the only option for some physical problems, such as heart or double-lung transplants. In this situation, the donor has passed away, but the organ is still healthy and able to function for years in the proper environment. In this situation, it is imperative that the donor organ be preserved, receiving proper oxygen and blood supply as long as possible before being transplanted. When this support is delayed, the organ can be irreversibly damaged.

Christian leaders in churches that have closed or ministries that have completed their intended goal still have much to contribute. In these situations, there is no risk of damage to the former ministry since it no longer functions. In these situations, the 'transplanted organ' is healthiest when they have continued in faithful ministry without long delays. Continual daily reliance on God more commonly dwindles as we relax in our ordinary lives, not actively ministering to others.

Donor Match

The key factor in any transplant is to find a good match. Several genetic markers are tested, the most obvious being blood type. As more of these markers are compatible, the risk of rejection is greatly reduced.

The early experiments in transplantation mentioned above occurred before knowledge of these markers was available. It seems ludicrous now to assume that an organ from a monkey or pig or goat could thrive in a human, and the results bear that out. The recipients never survived.

Interestingly, there was a recent news report about the transplantation of a genetically modified heart from a pig that occurred at the beginning of 2022. In this situation, there were no other options, and it was viewed as experimental. It required genetic modification of the donor material to remove the genetic markers identifying it as foreign tissue. Although this success was short-lived, time will tell if this is a viable source for patients with no other option.

In ministry, finding a good match to a difficult situation is vital. Stepping into the aftermath of leadership failure carries pressures and risks more than other leadership changes. The church board, as well as the denominational leadership (if available) must examine each candidate to see if they carry 'markers' of their ministry and personality that will promote healing in damaged circumstances.

God has promised He will build His Church, and the gates of hell will not overcome it. Thankfully, He will provide the leadership needed in each situation if we are just patient. After Jesus's ascension, the remaining disciples cast lots to find a replacement for Judas (Acts 1:23-26). This was, indeed, a failed leadership position, and they took it upon themselves to 'transplant' Matthias. And yet, he is not mentioned again in the bible. However, Saul of Tarsus seems to have been God's choice.

Patience in searching for the right 'transplant' is important, although in the interim, support of the hurting, damaged body is vital as well.

In 1 Kings 19, after the showdown on Mount Carmel, Elijah, in his despondence, felt he was alone in following God, yet God's still small voice assured him he had reserved seven thousand in Israel who had not fallen away (1 Kings 19:14, 18). In our pain, after surviving a great trial such as the failure of our leaders, we may feel alone and forsaken, but God is always present and preserves his servants. In the environment of hurting, lonely people, new leadership needs to share that still small voice of God to bring hope.

Rejection

Physically, transplanted organs are recognized as foreign tissue by the recipient. Variance in the genetic code between people leads to different markers that are then attacked by the immune system. This can lead to severe health issues and death if not addressed.

Through the years, various anti-rejection drugs have been developed to suppress this immune response. These are necessary for the successful acceptance of the new organ. Over time, tolerance to the new organ may improve, but medications are generally continued for life.

Use of these medications carries risk. Any medication that reduces the immune response increases the risk of infection since the immune system is our primary defense against invading germs. In addition, each individual medicine can have side effects in a variety of body systems.

Similarly, if a failing church receives a 'transplanted' pastor, rejection can occur. If the people, harmed by the moral failings of the departing leader, are hypersensitive or judgmental, this can harm the effectiveness of the new leadership. The best 'anti-rejection drug' in the church is the activity of the Holy Spirit. This fruit of love, joy, peace, longsuffering, kindness, goodness, faithfulness, gentleness, and self-control will provide support in an environment that promotes growth and healing to a hurting body.

Graft versus Host

A subtype of rejection is when the transplanted cells reject the new host body to which they were transplanted. This is usually a factor when the transplant provides immune function, such as bone marrow or stem cells. In this case, the immune cells in the newly transplanted bone marrow recognize the new host body as foreign with different genetic markers.

This graft vs host disease is widespread throughout all organs since the immune system circulates throughout the body. It can have a variety of symptoms as it attacks each tissue. The treatment still revolves around suppressing the immune response.

Spiritually, it is conceivable that a 'transplanted' leader to a new church will find the situation very difficult as they navigate the complications caused by the failure of their predecessor. In this situation, if the new leader rejects the church, damage is compounded and widespread. He may arrive with a judgmental tone and an aggressive ministry style, rejecting the good things that were already in place. Or he may clear out even humble supportive staff who have served for years through the pain of failed leadership.

It is true, this could be necessary for a fresh start, but he should strive to do this in a Godly way to avoid disrupting the ability of the church to move forward. Once again, the fruit of the Spirit is key to avoiding this type of rejection.

Like the physical body, as we reduce rejection spiritually, we sometimes go too far. We still must test everything and hold new leadership accountable, but if a church 'recipient' of a transplant relinquishes this duty to avoid conflict and to 'just get along,' false teaching could occur. Spiritual 'Infections' were discussed previously, and I will not repeat that here, but a church must continue to have discernment and seek God's guidance, especially in times of uncertainty and pain.

Summary

Organ transplantation is rarely desirable but sometimes necessary. In such dire circumstances, the life of the body is extended and strengthened, but will carry ongoing risks for both the recipient and the donor. In such situations, it is imperative to seek a good match before the transplant and to allow the fruit of the Spirit to permeate, reducing the risk of rejection. Then the body can continue to thrive and grow stronger.

What's in a name?

Our patient, Lynn Farmer, represents lymphoma, a cancer involving the lymphatic system. As described in this scenario, it generally is discovered when the patient or doctor notices an enlarging painless lymph node. Thankfully, many forms of lymphoma are successfully treated with surgery or chemotherapy, but some forms, as in our patient Lynn, are more aggressive and resistant to treatment. Although a large lymph node is one of the symptoms of this cancer, the majority of patient who come to the office concerned about lymph nodes will have nothing to worry about, and many times their worry about health issues is the primary problem we struggle to treat. And keep in mind that lymphoma has no relationship to a lipoma, a benign 'fatty tumor' of the skin.

Ends and Transitions

Our physical bodies are finite in their current form. Throughout this book, we have seen just a few of the afflictions we may face. Many heavy textbooks are filled with chapters describing innumerable conditions we risk in this fallen world. Even if we avoid most diseases and injuries that stalk us, our genetic programming includes a process called apoptosis, or programmed cell death. This is used to help destroy cells that may be problematic or are wearing out, and our tissues can produce new cells to replace them. Over time, this may play a part in aging and wasting away of tissues.

As various medical conditions accumulate, even the healthiest of us will still slow down and suffer some loss of ability. In 2 Corinthians 4:16, Paul tells us that as believers in Jesus, "…we do not lose heart. Even though our outward man is perishing, yet the inward man is being renewed day by day." Our suffering in this worldly existence, including the medical problems mentioned in the pages of this book, is referred to as "our light affliction, which is but for a moment" (verse 17) when we compare it to eternity.

Eventually, our health will fail, and we will die. The death rate is 100%. But, at the risk of sounding like a late-night infomercial, "Wait, there's more!" As believers, we know death is not the end. Just as a caterpillar enters the coffin-like cocoon only to be transformed into something unexpected and amazing, we will be transformed as well. Ecclesiastes 3:11 says, "He has made everything beautiful in its time. Also, He has put eternity in their hearts..." Maybe this refers to a blueprint for our glorified body embedded in our DNA.

Scripture tells us that when we die, our burial is like planting or sowing seed. Our physical "body is sown in corruption, it is raised in incorruption. It is sown in dishonor, it is raised in glory. It is sown in weakness, it is raised in power. It is sown a natural body, it is raised a spiritual body." (1 Corinthians 16:42-44).

We may not know exactly what our glorified body will be like, but there are some clues. After Jesus' resurrection, His glorified body was able to materialize in locked rooms and to disappear from the home of the travelers on the road to Emmaus. Yet, He was still recognizable to his disciples and was able to eat food. We also know that in heaven, in God's presence, "there shall be no more death, nor sorrow, nor crying. There shall be no more pain, for the former things have passed away." (Revelation 21:4). How awesome that will be!

How does this apply to the Body of Christ? The Bible does not have many clear statements about the church in Heaven. Hebrews says:

> But you have come to Mount Zion and to the city of the living God, the heavenly Jerusalem, to an innumerable company of angels, to the general assembly and **church of the firstborn** who are registered in heaven, to God the Judge of all, to the spirits of just men made perfect, to Jesus the Mediator of the new covenant". (Hebrews 12:22-24, emphasis mine).

Here on earth, the church as the Body of Christ is His representation to the world. We minister to those who are hurting, we reach the lost, sharing the good news of salvation, and we stand as a beacon, shedding light in a dark world. In heaven, it seems to me that the church in this form will no longer be needed. Glory will be filled with 'just men made perfect,' and Jesus will be there in person. There will not be unsaved people, nor will there be pain and suffering.

As for shedding light in darkness, Revelation 22:5 tells us: "There shall be no night there: They need no lamp nor light of the sun, for the Lord God gives them light."

So what does this mean for the church? Perhaps it will be transformed into something unforeseen. It seems our physical bodies will be transformed, shedding some of the functions and adaptations that allow us to fight illness, survive in times of distress, and repair damage from disease, leaving us free to truly live unencumbered. We will enjoy true health as God intended at creation.

Similarly, the church, as the earthly representation of the Body of Christ, will be set free to be the glorious church without spot or wrinkle that God intended. We may experience perfect fellowship without friction or strife and participate in true worship as it was intended. This perfection of the church is referred to in scripture as being the Bride of Christ. In our physical bodies, the bride and groom sharing intimacy become one flesh. In the spiritual realm, the Bride of Christ and the Bridegroom, Jesus, share deep intimacy that leads to being one in spirit.

Imagine the best church service you have been in, experiencing God's presence and the working of the Holy Spirit. On earth, those experiences seem to fade quickly as we go to work the next morning or face hard things. But once we reach heaven, we will be continually in His presence and will worship with the angels. We will be 'the church of the firstborn' as quoted above.

The end of our existence on earth is not really the end. Both as a physical body and as the Body of Christ, we will be transformed. Our temporal existence provides us with a limited understanding of the eternal. C. S. Lewis described it as imagining someone living in a two-dimensional world, like a flat piece of paper, trying to understand what a three-dimensional object must be like. He would know a square as four lines, but a cube would be six of those squares at right angles to each other. He would have no concept of height, only of length and width, therefore, unable to visualize a cube. Maybe heaven is like a six- or eight-dimensional place (or more), far beyond our ability to comprehend. (Lewis goes into more detail in his sermon/essay entitled 'Transposition,' published in "The Weight of Glory and other addresses," copyright 1975, Touchstone books, pp 72-89).

In the meantime, we live here on earth, eagerly longing for His coming. While we continue on as members of the Body of Christ, we have a responsibility to our fellow "Body parts" to, first of all, keep ourselves spiritually healthy, but secondly, to build them up as well. In Ephesians 4, Paul tells us God appointed various spiritual roles in the Body of Christ, including apostles, prophets, evangelists, pastors, and teachers. The reason for this is to promote the health of the Body. As Paul wrote in one amazing sentence, God provided spiritual gifts to each of us:

> "for the equipping of the saints for the work of ministry, for the edifying of the body of Christ, till we all come to the unity of the faith and of the knowledge of the Son of God, to a perfect man, to the measure of the stature of the fullness of Christ; that we should no longer be children, tossed to and fro and carried about with every wind of doctrine, by the trickery of men, in the cunning craftiness of deceitful plotting, but, speaking the truth in love, may grow up in all things into Him who is the head—Christ—from whom the whole body, joined and knit together by what every joint supplies, according to the effective working by

which every part does its share, causes growth of the body for the edifying of itself in love." Ephesians 4:12-16

Throughout this book, I have pointed out some of the possible problems we may face individually and as a church. My hope is that we will recognize them early, in the beginning stages, so we can do our part in edifying the body.

Remember, as members of the Body, we need to grow up and be joined together, contributing to the health of the Church. We must each do our share, and that is how the Body can thrive.

Most importantly, all of this is to be done in love.

Appendix**
(Why is this even here?)

Problem 1.

Aiden borrows a book from the public library. He reads a few pages on day one. On day two, he reads twice the number of pages that he read on day one. On the third day, he reads six pages less than what he read on the first day. If he has read the entire book that contains 458 pages, how many pages did he read on day three?

Problem 2.

A math limerick:

A dozen, a gross, and a score

Plus three times the square root of four

Divided by seven
Plus five times eleven
Is [ ] and not a bit more.

Problem 3.

You walk up to a mountain that has two paths. One leads to the other side of the mountain, and the other will get you lost forever. Two twins know the path that leads to the other side. You can ask them only one question. Except! One lies and one tells the truth, and you don't know which is which. So, what do you ask?

Problem 4.

In your cellar, there are three light switches in the OFF position. Each switch controls one of three light bulbs on the floor above it. You may move any of the switches, but you may only go upstairs to inspect the bulbs one time. How can you find the switch for each bulb with one inspection?

Answers on the next page.

**** If your appendix gives you problems, you may remove it, being very careful to not harm the rest of the body (of the book)**

Answers

1. Answer: 110.

   Day one he reads 'A' pages. Day 2, he reads 'A' x 2, Day 3, 'A' - 6.

   Total pages = (A)+(2A)+(A-6)=458
   4A-6 = 458
   4A=464
   A=116 (the number of pages read on day one)

Since on day 3 he reads A-6 pages, that would be 116 - 6=110. (from http://mathworksheets4kids.com/equations/word-problems/multi-step-integers1.pdf)

2. Answer: Nine Squared.

12 +144+20		= 176
Plus 3 x 2	+6	=182
Divided by 7		=26
Plus 55		=81 (aka nine squared.)

(Heard on the "Car Talk" radio program as one of their 'puzzlers.' Date unknown)

3. Answer: You ask each twin 'What would your brother say?.' Let's say the correct path is on the left side. If you asked the liar, "What would your brother say?" The liar would know his brother was honest, and he would say the left side, but since the liar lies, he would say right. If you asked the honest twin the same question, he would say right, because

he knows his brother will lie. Therefore, you would know that the correct path was the left.

(found at http://solveordie.com/riddle-263/)

4. Answer: Number the switches 1,2, and 3. Switch on number 1 for one minute, then switch it off. Switch on number 2 and go upstairs.

   The light that is on is connected to switch 2. The light that is off and warm is connected to switch 1. The light that is off and cold is connected to switch 3!

   (found at https://www.mathsisfun.com/cellar_problem_solution.html)

www.ingramcontent.com/pod-product-compliance
Lightning Source LLC
LaVergne TN
LVHW022042200926
848481LV00003B/758
* 9 7 9 8 9 9 4 2 3 0 6 8 8 *